Arrhythmia Management in Chagas' Disease

edited by

Maria Cristina Tentori, M.D.

Chief of Electrophysiology and Pacing
Juan A. Fernandez Hospital
Buenos Aires, Argentina

Elsa L. Segura, M.D.

Director of the Administración Nacional de Laboratorios e
Institutos de Salud (ANLIS)
Dr. Carlos G. Malbran, Ministerio de Salud y Acción
Social
Member of the Research Center of CONICET
Argentina

David L. Hayes, M.D.

Consultant, Division of Cardiovascular Diseases and
Internal Medicine
Mayo Clinic and Mayo Foundation
Professor of Medicine, Mayo Medical School
Rochester, Minnesota

Futura Publishing Company, Inc.
Armonk, NY

Library of Congress Cataloging-in-Publication Data

Arrhythmia management in Chagas' disease / editors, Maria
Cristina Tentori, Elsa L. Segura, Hayes, David L.
   p. cm.
  Includes bibliographical references and index.
  ISBN 0-87993-450-6 (hardcover : alk. paper)
   1. Arrhythmia. 2. Chagas' disease—Complications. I. Tentori,
Maria Cristina. II. Segura, Elsa L. III. Hayes, David L.

RC685.A65 A772 2000
616.1'28—dc21

                                99-053035

Published by
Futura Publishing Company, Inc.
135 Bedford Road
Armonk, NY 10504-0418

ISBN# 0-87993-450-6

Every effort has been made to ensure that the information in this book
is as up-to-date and as accurate as possible at the time of publication.
However, due to the constant developments in medicine, neither the
author, nor the editor, nor the publisher can accept any legal or any
other responsibility for any errors or omissions that may occur.

Printed in the United States of America.
This book is printed on acid-free paper.

Contributors

Harry Acquatella, M.D., F.A.C.C.
Professor, Faculty of Medicine, U.C.V.-Hospital Universitario de Caracas

Pablo A. Chiale, M.D.
Chief, In-Patients Ward, Division of Cardiology, Ramos Mejía Hospital, Buenos Aires, Argentina

André d'Avila, M.D.
Assistant of the Arrhythmias Clinical Unit of the Heart Institute, University of São Paulo, Brazil

Marcelo V. Elizari, M.D., F.A.C.C., F.A.H.A.
Chief, Division of Cardiology, Ramos Mejía Hospital, Buenos Aires, Argentina

Hugo Giordano, M.D.
Professor, Faculty of Medicine, U.C.V.-Hospital Universitario de Caracas

Cidio Halperin, M.D.
Director, Electrophysiology Services, Hospital São Francisco and Hospital Ernesto Dornelles, Porto Alegre, Brazil

David L. Hayes, M.D.
Consultant, Division of Cardiovascular Diseases and Internal Medicine, Mayo Clinic and Mayo Foundation; Professor of Medicine, Mayo Medical School; Rochester, Minnesota

Mariano J. Levin, M.D.
Laboratorio de Biología Molecular de la Enfermedad de Chagas-INGEBI, Buenos Aires, Argentina

José Gregorio Loyo, M.D.
Centro Médico de Caracas

Cristián Madoery, M.D.
Staff, Electrophysiology and Pacing, Juan A. Fernandez Hospital, Buenos Aires, Argentina

Roberto Madoery, M.D.
Hospital Privado, Córdoba, Argentina

Antonio Martínez-Rubio, M.D.
Hospital Sant Pau i Sant Creu, Barcelona, Spain

iii

Carlos A. Morillo, M.D.
Professor, Department of Medicine, Universidad Industrial de Santander, Chairman, Department of Cardiology and Cardiovascular Sciences, Director, Laboratory of Autonomic Physiology, Fundación Cardiovascular del Oriente Colombiano Instituto del Corazón, Bucaramanga, Santander, Colombia

Claudio Muratore, M.D.
Sanatorio Mitre, Buenos Aires, Argentina

Juan José Puigbó, M.D., F.A.C.C.
Professor, Faculty of Medicine, U.C.V.-Hospital Universitario de Caracas

Rafael Rabinovich, M.D.
Sanatorio Mitre, Buenos Aires, Argentina

Sergio Rassi, M.D.
Professor of Cardiology, School of Medicine, Federal University of Goias, Goiania, Brazil, Chief, Electrophysiology and Arrhythmias Division, Sao Salvador Hospital, Goiania, Goias

Aurora Ruiz, M.D.
Juan A. Fernandez Hospital, Buenos Aires, Argentina

Mauricio Scanavacca, M.D.
Associate Professor of Cardiology and Assistant of the Arrhythmias Clinical Unit of the Heart Institute, University of São Paulo, Brazil

Elsa L. Segura, M.D.
Director of the Administración Nacional de Laboratorios e Institutos de Salud (ANLIS) Dr. Carlos G. Malbran, Ministerio de Salud y Acción Social and Member of the Research Center of CONICET, Argentina

Eduardo Sosa, M.D.
Associated Professor of Cardiology and Director of the Arrhythmias Clinical Unit of the Heart Institute, University of São Paulo, Brazil

Claudia Suárez, M.D.
Professor, Faculty of Medicine, U.C.V.-Instituto de Anatomia Patológica

Maria Cristina Tentori, M.D.
Chief of Electrophysiology and Pacing, Juan A. Fernandez Hospital, Buenos Aires, Argentina

Claudio de Zuloaga, M.D.
Electrophysiology Laboratory, Posadas Hospital, Buenos Aires, Argentina

Preface

Most clinicians in the United States know little about Chagas' disease other than that it occurs in South and Central America. As a cardiologist practicing in the Midwest region of the United States, before I embarked on this project I knew only this and the fact that Chagas' disease is the most common cause of atrioventricular block in South America.

Unorthodox as it may be, it is necessary that I begin this text with an explanation of how the project evolved and why I am involved. A book editor is generally selected, whether by oneself or not, because of extensive experience in the field and, often, having published widely on the subject. Because I have never seen a patient with Chagas' disease, or at least one that I've recognized, and have never published on Chagas' disease, my participation in this project must be justified.

One of the rewards of working and publishing in the field of cardiac pacing has been to become familiar with the Latin American pacing and electrophysiology community and to develop close friends throughout this region of the world. Talking with many Latin American colleagues about the difficulties and frustrations encountered in treating arrhythmias associated with Chagas' disease stimulated an interest in the subject, even if it was one that most likely would never be applicable to my practice or research. Newer applications of pacing and implantable cardioverter-defibrillator therapy have potential promise for application to patients with Chagas' disease. Limitation of the necessary technology and the ability to finance and carry out clinical trials in Latin American countries frustrates not only experts in electrophysiology and Chagas' disease in those countries but also physicians who observe from elsewhere. Those of us who know the Latin American pacing and electrophysiology community are aware of the individual and collective expertise that exists and the additional contributions that could be made in many areas of pacing and electrophysiology, especially in a disease that is endemic to several of their countries, that is, Chagas' disease.

As plans were made for an international meeting on pacing, electrophysiology, and arrhythmia management to be held in South America, it seemed an excellent time to bring together experts from several Latin American countries to prepare this text. Dr. Tentori, Dr. Segura, and

I recognize that there are many experts on Chagas' disease throughout Central and South America. In a monograph of limited size, only a limited number of contributors could be included. Although we apologize to those experts who have not been included, we believe that we have collected excellent information from multiple experts that will add to the understanding and management of arrhythmias in the patient with Chagas' disease.

—David L. Hayes, M.D.

Introduction

Chagas' disease, or trypanosomiasis cruzi, is an endemic disease that ranks third in both prevalence and incidence in Latin America. According to reports, this disease causes 45 thousand deaths yearly due to cardiopathy and is one of the pathologic conditions with the highest index of unpredictable sudden death. Socioeconomic implications should be pointed out, since this disease has been traditionally related to poverty. Migration of this population with low economic resources occurred within the same country or between neighboring countries. Perhaps this is one of the reasons why this disease has been limited to and is pathognomonic of Latin America.

Currently, with globalization and macroeconomics, the poverty zones are increasingly larger, and this expansion may be responsible for important migratory movements to faraway places in the search for new horizons and income sources. We should bear in mind that a high percentage of the chagasic population consists of young persons in working activities.

I am pleased to announce that this book contains the efforts of a number of contributors from different countries in South America. I believe that the prospect of unifying both the effort and the experience of colleagues who are dealing with Chagas' disease and arrhythmia is very important. I hope the reader finds that we have succeeded in the attempt to provide brief but complete information about arrhythmia in Chagas' myocardiopathy and its treatment.

I thank Futura Publishing for supporting this book, the talented contributors for their effort and enthusiasm, and last but not least, Dr. David Hayes for creating this project and giving full support.

As a concluding statement, and so far only as a wish, I encourage all Latin American governments to make a real commitment and join efforts with world organizations to eradicate this disease.

—Maria Cristina Tentori, M.D.

Contents

Preface
    David L. Hayes v

Introduction
    Maria Cristina Tentori 7

1. Chagas' Heart Disease in the United States
    David L. Hayes 1

2. Etiology, Pathophysiology, and Diagnosis of Chagas' Disease
    Elsa L. Segura 5

3. Molecular Pathology of Chagas' Disease
    Mariano J. Levin 19

4. Clinical Aspects of Chagas' Disease
    Juan José Puigbó, Harry Acquatella, Claudia Suárez, José Gregorio Loyo,
    Hugo Giordano 27

5. Effects of Chagas' Disease on Cardiac Autonomic Reflex Function
    Carlos A. Morillo 51

6. Signal-Averaged Electrocardiography in Chagas' Disease
    Cristián Madoery, Aurora Ruiz, Antonio Martínez-Rubio,
    Roberto Madoery 67

7. Clinical Relevance of Invasive Electrophysiologic Studies in Patients
    With Chagas' Disease
    Cidio Halperin, Sérgio Rassi 83

8. Pharmacologic Treatment of Arrhythmias Related to Chronic Chagas'
    Heart Disease
    Marcelo V. Elizari, Pablo A. Chiale 95

9. Surgery and Catheter Ablation for the Treatment of Ventricular
    Tachycardia in Chagas' Disease
    Eduardo Sosa, Mauricio Scanavacca, André d'Avila 117

10. Use of the Implantable Cardioverter-Defibrillator in Chagas' Disease
    Claudio Muratore, Rafael Rabinovich 129

11. Bradyarrhythmias in Chagasic Cardiomyopathy
    Claudio de Zuloaga 143

Chapter 1

Chagas' Heart Disease in the United States

David L. Hayes, M.D.

An article by Hagar and Rahimtoola[1] provides an excellent and complete overview of Chagas' heart disease in the United States as assessed in the 1990s. The authors conclude that Chagas' heart disease is being encountered with increasing frequency in North America, predominantly in persons immigrating to the United States from Central American countries. They estimate that between 400,000 and 500,000 persons residing in the United States are infected with *Trypanosoma cruzi*. Kirchhoff[2] estimated in 1993 that there were 50,000 to 100,000 immigrants with *T. cruzi* living in the United States. This estimate was based on a study of 205 Nicaraguan and Salvadoran immigrants living in Washington, D.C., 5% of whom were found to be infected.

As other chapters in this monograph reflect, the clinical manifestations of Chagas' heart disease may be diverse, increasing the difficulty of diagnosis. Diagnosis is especially difficult in a country such as the United States, where the rarity of the disease along with the diverse manifestations may lead to misdiagnosis or nonrecognition of the disease state. An editorial in the *American Heart Journal*[3] considered whether Chagas' disease exists as an undiagnosed form of cardiomyopathy. Experts from the Centro de Enfermedad de Chagas in Buenos Aires and from the pathology branch of the National Heart, Lung, and Blood Institute estimated that 74,000 Latin Americans living in the United States had chronic chagasic cardiomyopathy. They went on to state that the cardiomyopathy was either not diagnosed or misdiagnosed as idiopathic dilated cardiomyopathy or coronary artery disease.

Regardless of the exact number of persons living in the United States who are infected with *T. cruzi*, the concern is whether the prevalence of the disease in North American countries will increase as a

From Tentori MC, Segura EL, Hayes DL (eds.) *Arrhythmia Management in Chagas' Disease*. Armonk, NY: Futura Publishing Co., Inc. ©2000.

result of larger numbers of presumably infected immigrants. Milei et al.[3] pointed out that variations in the biologic behavior of North American species of insect vectors and a difference in living conditions make the traditional vector transmission of the disease unlikely. Instead, they expressed the belief that blood transfusion from infected but asymptomatic patients would be the most likely avenue of transmission of the disease. This subject has been considered in other contemporary publications.[4-6]

In a study specifically designed to determine the prevalence of antibodies to *T. cruzi*, 6,013 randomly selected serum samples from the southeastern United States were tested.[5] Only 10 of the samples were positive by one or more methods, a result suggesting that although parasites and vectors are found in the southeastern United States and that both infect mammals,[7,8] the risk of infection to humans in this region is negligible. Despite this encouraging study, case reports of Chagas' disease in southern states have emerged.[9,10]

In an effort to screen potential blood donors, Appleman et al.[6] created a questionnaire to identify donors who may be at high risk for *T. cruzi* infection. After a brief description of Chagas' disease, the questionnaire continues with the following nine questions:

1. Were you born in, have you lived in, or have you traveled to Central America, South America, or southeastern Mexico?
2. Have you ever been told that you had Chagas' disease or a positive test for Chagas' disease?

If the answer to Question 1 or 2 is yes, please answer all of the following questions.

3. Have you ever slept in a home or building with a palm leaf-thatched roof and/or walls made of mud?
4. Have you had a blood transfusion or shots of blood while in Latin America?
5. Do you have an enlarged heart?
6. Do you have an abnormal heart rhythm?
7. Do you have gastrointestinal problems?
8. Have you ever had an unexplained illness with fevers?
9. Have you ever had facial swelling while in or shortly after a visit to Latin America?

Although the incidence of Chagas' disease does not appear to be increasing in North America at an alarming rate, the disease clearly exists in the immigrant population and the incidence has the potential to increase via blood transfusions. Recommendations from North American colleagues[1,11] as well as the information provided in this book should help the interested clinician in managing chagasic heart disease and, specifically, the arrhythmic manifestations of Chagas' disease.

Currently, there is great interest in the application of biventricular or left ventricular pacing in patients with congestive heart failure secondary to ischemic or dilated cardiomyopathy. In addition, cardioverter-defibrillator implantation for primary prevention of sudden death has stimulated much interest and continuing clinical trials. The therapeutic usefulness of a device that combines biventricular pacing and cardioverter-defibrillator therapy is also undergoing evaluation in various parts of the world. Therapy with such a device would seem to have extraordinary potential for patients with Chagas' heart disease.

It is hoped that this book along with the preexisting interest of many highly qualified Latin American experts in pacing and electrophysiology will stimulate not only the rest of the clinical community but also governmental and commercial organizations to finance and participate in research and clinical trials necessary to improve the therapeutic options for patients with Chagas' heart disease.

References

1. Hagar JM, Rahimtoola SH: Chagas' heart disease in the United States. N Engl J Med 325:763-768, 1991
2. Kirchhoff LV: American trypanosomiasis (Chagas' disease)—a tropical disease now in the United States. N Engl J Med 329:639-644, 1993
3. Milei J, Mautner B, Storino R, Sanches JA, Ferrans VJ: Does Chagas' disease exist as an undiagnosed form of cardiomyopathy in the United States? Am Heart J 123:1732-1735, 1992
4. Wendel S, Gonzaga AL: Chagas' disease and blood transfusion: a new world problem? Vox Sang 64:1-12, 1993
5. Barrett VJ, Leiby DA, Odom JL, Otani MM, Rowe JD, Roote JT, Cox KF, Brown KR, Hoiles JA, Saez-Alquézar A, Turrens JF: Negligible prevalence of antibodies against *Trypanosoma cruzi* among blood donors in the southeastern United States. Am J Clin Pathol 108:499-503, 1997
6. Appleman IA, Shulman SS, Kirchhoff LV: Use of a questionnaire to identify potential blood donors at risk for infection with *Trypanosoma cruzi*. Transfusion 33:61-64, 1993
7. Pietrzak SM, Pung OJ: Trypanosomiasis in raccoons from Georgia. J Wildl Dis 34:132-136, 1998
8. Barr SC, Gossett KA, Klei TR: Clinical, clinicopathologic, and parasitologic observations of trypanosomiasis in dogs infected with North American *Trypanosoma cruzi* isolates. Am J Vet Res 52:954-960, 1991
9. Cimo PL, Luper WE, Scouros MA: Transfusion-associated Chagas' disease in Texas: report of a case. Tex Med 89:48-50, 1993
10. Holbert RD, Magiros E, Hirsch CP, Nunenmacher SJ: Chagas' disease: a case in south Mississippi. J Miss State Med Assoc 36:1-5, 1995
11. Acquatella H, Schiller NB: Echocardiographic recognition of Chagas' disease and endomyocardial fibrosis. J Am Soc Echocardiogr 1:60-68, 1988

Chapter 2

Etiology, Pathophysiology, and Diagnosis of Chagas' Disease

Elsa L. Segura, M.D.

Etiology of Chagas' Disease and Transmission of *Trypanosoma cruzi*

Among the 80 so-called tropical diseases, Chagas' disease ranks as one of the most important public health problems on the American continent. From Argentina and Chile to Mexico, approximately 16 million people are infected with *T. cruzi*.[1] Chagas' disease, or American trypanosomiasis, is a parasitic disease produced by *Trypanosoma (Schizotrypanum) cruzi* (phylum, Protozoa; superclass, Mastigophora; order, Kinetoplastida). The life cycle of *T. cruzi* alternates between a mammal host and an insect vector. From a public health perspective, vector-mediated transmission of *T. cruzi* is still the most important mode of transmission, followed by infection through blood transfusion, infected women to offspring, and organ transplantation.[1] Congenital disease can be detected by serologic and parasitologic methods within the first year of life and, if treated at an early age, the patient can be cured.[2] Accidental, some even fatal, laboratory infections by *T. cruzi* and infections during surgical procedures have been reported.[3,4]

T. cruzi has different physiologic and morphologic stages characterized by the position of the flagellum and kinetoplast relative to the cell nucleus.[5] No antigenic variation of *T. cruzi* has been demonstrated, nor have highly immunodominant antigens, as in other protozoa, been described to date. The parasites multiply extracellularly as epimastigotes in the intestine of triatomine bugs and develop to metacyclic trypomastigotes in the rectal ampule, from which they are excreted

From Tentori MC, Segura EL, Hayes DL (eds.) *Arrhythmia Management in Chagas' Disease.* Armonk, NY: Futura Publishing Co., Inc. ©2000.

with feces.[6] When triatomines defecate during and immediately after blood feeding, the trypomastigotes are excreted around the area bitten by the insect. This placement and the subsequent itching favor the penetration of trypomastigotes into the mammal host tissues.[7] Trypomastigotes are able to infect a variety of host cells once they penetrate the skin cells or the mucous membranes.

The mechanism of infection has been studied in cell cultures and is essentially the same in all cases: An active process, most likely involving chemotactic substances produced by the host, allows the trypomastigote to reach the cell cytoplasm and differentiate into an amastigote form.[8] After reproducing by binary fission, amastigotes differentiate again into trypomastigotes, destroy the host cell, and escape into the interstitial space or the bloodstream several days after infection.[4] Trypomastigotes can reach any part of the body and invade other cells, especially the muscular fibers or the reticuloendothelial cells. The circulating trypomastigotes close the transmission cycle when a triatomine bug sucks the blood of an infected person with parasitemia. The infected bug then transmits metacyclic trypomastigotes to a susceptible host. A portion (15% to 30%) of infected persons have symptoms that characterize the chronic stage of the disease.[1,3,9] The etiology of the Chagas' disease lesion is widely attributed to *T. cruzi* and heart involvement, as demonstrated in all 58 acute cases of Chagas' disease detected in western Venezuela from 1989 to 1997.[10]

Pathophysiology of Chagas' Disease

One of the hallmarks of Chagas' disease is the cardiomyopathy that develops in the chronic stage of infection.[3] The pathogenesis of chronic myocarditis associated with *T. cruzi* is not well understood. Most studies on the pathogenesis of Chagas' disease have been directed to determine the role of the parasite and the various arms of the host immune system in relation to infection and disease development. Cellular and humoral responses have been extensively studied in relation to their participation in the immune response to *T. cruzi* and in the development of chronic chagasic myocarditis.

The correlation between an effective immune response and control of infection has been well established. Impairment of the immune system usually results in disease that is more severe. The predominance of CD8+ T lymphocytes and production of various cytokines in the inflammatory sites strongly indicate their active role in the host immune response to infection.[11] Various studies have also demonstrated the trypanocidal capabilities of interferon-γ-activated macrophages mediated by nitric oxide. The administration of nitric oxide inhibitors to mice infected with *T. cruzi* further demonstrated the role of this molecule in the natural resistance to the parasite.

Nitric oxide produced by activated macrophages is also known to be cytotoxic for a variety of other intracellular pathogens, including

Leishmania major, Toxoplasma gondii, Schistosoma mansoni, and *T. cruzi.* In addition, the role of the immune response elicited by *T. cruzi* in the development of heart disease remains unclear.

Autoimmunity has been proposed as a major mechanism accounting for the cardiac lesions, mainly because of the low number of parasites detected in patients with chronic chagasic disease and the occurrence of antibodies reacting with both *T. cruzi* and human tissues.[12] However, with the development of new techniques for the identification of subcellular fractions of microorganisms, various authors have demonstrated the relation between *T. cruzi* components and the development of heart disease.[11,13] In addition, specific anti-*T. cruzi* treatment has been shown to result in a more favorable clinical prognosis for the disease.[14] These findings strongly indicate that the persistence of parasites is a major determinant for the progression of disease.

Diagnosis of *T. cruzi* Infection in Different Clinical and Epidemiologic Settings

The parasite or some of its components and the antibodies against *T. cruzi* are important for assessing clinical and chemotherapeutic progress and the effect of control actions on *T. cruzi* transmission. In vector-mediated transmission, one method of surveillance is the serologic follow-up of seronegative children since the beginning of insecticidal spraying activities; new infections are demonstrated through seroconversion.[15] The detection of infected pregnant women and follow-up of their newborn infants are also accomplished by serologic and parasitologic methods.[2] Donated blood is controlled through serologic methods.

T. cruzi is nearly always found in the bloodstream during the first 10 weeks after infection in patients experiencing the acute phase. A drop of fresh blood between slide and cover slip is examined microscopically at x400. Thin and thick blood smears are also recommended. These simple methods allow detection of *T. cruzi* in approximately 71% of patients.[16] The Strout method is the simplest, allowing identification of *T. cruzi* in 95% of acute cases.[17] This method has been adapted for application to nursing newborns by taking a blood sample in four capillary tubes[18] and can be used for detecting *T. cruzi* in cerebrospinal fluid.

The indirect parasitologic methods used are xenodiagnosis, hemoculture, and animal inoculation. Xenodiagnosis takes advantage of the multiplication of *T. cruzi* in the vector.[19,20] Uninfected *Triatoma infestans* third or fourth instar nymphs reared in the laboratory on birds, which are refractory to *T. cruzi* infection, are applied to the patient's legs or arms for 20 to 30 minutes. Ten *T. infestans* bugs are used in infants below 1 year of age, 20 bugs are used in children from 2 to 12 years old, and 40 bugs are used in patients older than 13. The sensitivity of xenodiagnosis is 100% for acute disease and 50% for chronic infection. Achieving these sensitivity values requires microscopic examination of each cover slip for 30 minutes.[20] Natural and artificial xenodiagnosis in seroreactive patients yielded very similar results when *Dipetalogaster maximus* first instar nymphs were used.[21] A statistically significant inverse association between age and parasitemia in patients seroreactive for *T. cruzi* has been reported by several authors.[22,23]

Hemoculture has also been used extensively, because *T. cruzi* is easily cultured in axenic media containing haemine or its derivatives.[24] Procedures with different treatment of the patient's blood or different composition of culture media have been tried extensively.[24-26] Hemoculture repeated at least twice has a 50% sensitivity in detecting *T. cruzi* in patients during the chronic or indeterminate phase.[27] Moreover, in 59 acute-phase cases studied in Venezuela, the more sensitive parasitologic methods were xenodiagnosis and hemoculture.[28] Animal inoculation is also used to isolate the parasite when parasitemia is scanty or when an organ transplant from a *T. cruzi*-infected donor is needed.[29]

Because the intensity of parasitemia is low during the indeterminate and chronic phases, serologic methods are needed for detecting *T. cruzi* infection. The sensitivity of the serologic methods depends on the immunologic response of the host to *T. cruzi* infection. Despite different profiles of infection among patients, specific IgM to *T. cruzi* antigens is detected 1 week after infection, peaks at 30 days, and decreases to undetectable levels 3 to 4 months after infection, when IgG antibodies reach their maximum expression. Low levels of specific IgM detected in different phases of the disease are not associated with any specific clinical feature. Specific IgG reaches the highest concentration 4 to 6 weeks after infection.[30] When patients with acute or indeterminate disease are treated, different degrees of negativization occur.[14,31] Rare cases of spontaneous reversion to a seronegative status without specific chemotherapy have been described.[32]

The antibodies against *T. cruzi* can be detected by several methods. The usefulness of these methods and their application depends on the epidemiologic context and the human and technical resources available to the health services. Quality control of antigen preparation lots and laboratory procedures is crucially needed.[33]

Serologic methods have been applied to field animal populations to assess the relative importance of reservoir species and the efficacy of vector control actions. An enzyme-linked immunosorbent assay (ELISA) for detecting specific anti-*T. cruzi* antibodies was standardized and compared with other routine techniques. In adult dogs naturally infected with *T. cruzi*, as determined by a positive xenodiagnosis, sensitivity was 94% for both ELISA and the indirect fluorescent antibody test.[34]

A complement fixation test detected antibodies against *T. cruzi* 4 weeks after infection.[35] Direct agglutination is performed with a suspension of formalin-fixed epimastigotes of *T. cruzi*.[36] A particle gel immunoassay was developed in which red particles are sensitized with three synthetic peptides representing antigen sequences of *T. cruzi*.[37]

For quantitative indirect hemagglutination assays, the antigen is the supernatant of disrupted (compression-decompression) epimastigotes centrifuged at 10,000g and preserved by lyophilization.[38,39] The lyophilized antigen is incubated with sheep or chicken red blood cells treated with tannic acid. The sensitized red blood cells are then used as antigen and incubated with the test serum. The reaction is performed in duplicate in microtiter plates with a fixed dilution of the sensitized red blood cells. Reactivity is revealed by a film covering 50% to 100% of the bottom of the well. The indirect hemagglutination assay, evaluated with serum panels in various reference centers, has a sensitivity and specificity of approximately 99% and 98%, respectively.[40] The indirect hemagglutination assay was the most specific and sensitive test in a recent study in blood banks in Brazil[41] and is widely used in routine work.

The indirect immunofluorescence reaction uses as antigen epimastigotes from axenic cultures treated with formaldehyde and fixed in glass smears that can be maintained for several months at −20°C.[42,43] The antigen-antibody complex is revealed with anti-human fluorescein-labeled IgG by use of serial serum dilutions. This method has a high sensitivity (98% to 99%) and specificity.

The ELISA has been successful in detecting antigens and antibodies against several infectious diseases.[44] Several immunoenzymatic assays with different antigens, ranging from *T. cruzi* recombinant protein mixtures and synthetic molecules to proteins or peptides, are being used for serodiagnosis of *T. cruzi* infection. Six *T. cruzi* recombinant antigens were evaluated by ELISA in 541 sera of reactive and nonreactive patients from nine Central and South American[45] countries in a multicenter study. Sensitivity was 79% to 100%, and specificity ranged from 96.2% to 99.6%. With epimastigote crude antigens, however, the specificity was only 84%.

Use of a combination of recombinant antigens has been proposed.[45] A radioimmunoprecipitation-confirmed assay combining a tripeptide and three epitopes in an ELISA confirmed that the combination of peptides containing multiple repeat epitopes is a powerful means of detecting anti-*T. cruzi* antibodies.[46] A field study of the immune response to the shed acute phase antigen (SAPA) of *T. cruzi* showed that the anti-SAPA response not only is present during the initial acute stage of the infection (a few months) but also extends some years after infection.[47] Another procedure suggested for the acute phase uses an 80-kd *T. cruzi* antigen, which is eliminated in the urine of infected hosts during the acute stage. Human antibodies to urinary antigens immunoprecipitated this *T. cruzi* antigen and also inhibited the binding of the monoclonal antibody to the urinary antigen in an inhibition assay.[48]

Immunoblotting with trypomastigote excreted-secreted antigens (TESA blot) of *T. cruzi* has been evaluated as a diagnostic method for chronic, acute, and congenital Chagas' disease. Serum samples from acute-phase and congenital infections were considered to be positive when they reacted with ladder-like bands of 130- to 200-kd antigens recognized by IgM and IgG antibodies, whereas IgG from chronic-phase sera recognized a broad-band antigen of 150 to 160 kd.[49]

Molecular Methods for Diagnosis of *T. cruzi* Infection

One of the main problems facing diagnosis is the heterogeneity of *T. cruzi* in the Americas. Schizodeme analysis is based on the comparison of electrophoretic patterns of kinetoplast DNA restriction fragments and can be an adequate means of parasite characterization because of its sensitivity.[50-52] One of its limitations stems from the possibility of selecting parasite subpopulations. As in zymodeme analysis, the number of different schizodeme patterns is virtually identical to the number of parasite isolates. This phenomenon led some authors to suggest a multiclonal structure for *T. cruzi* and raised the question of whether the difference between patterns could reflect evolution times between strains.[53,54]

In *T. cruzi* infection, the polymerase chain reaction (PCR) is important for the diagnosis of immunologic compromise and for assessment of the effects of drug treatment. PCR may also be used to detect parasites in the feces of triatomine bugs and thus to obtain more accurate results in xenodiagnosis and entomologic surveys in endemic areas. Previous studies of PCR in the detection of *T. cruzi* used genomic DNA, kDNA, nuclear intergenic ribosomal DNA,[51] and ribosomal RNA.[55-59] A PCR with the nuclear primers bp1/bp2 has been used to detect *T. cruzi* DNA in the blood of infected patients and feces of triatomine bugs; specificity and sensitivity are high.[60]

A PCR technique was compared with hemoculture or complement-mediated lysis in 113 persons from endemic areas of Brazil who had conventional serologic results scored as positive, negative, or inconclusive.[61] The PCR results were positive in many persons with seronegative or serologically inconclusive findings and negative in all uninfected control subjects. Perhaps the installation of a quality assurance program[33] for serodiagnosis will increase the accuracy of serodiagnosis in comparison with that of PCR. In another study, the approximately 330-bp fragment of the kinetoplast minicircles was used as a target for amplification. The use of chemiluminescence on slot blots with a specific alkaline phosphatase–conjugated oligonucleotide probe detected specific products from as little as 0.1 pg of *T. cruzi* kDNA.[62] PCR was successfully used to detect *T. cruzi* in dried feces of *T. infestans*[60,63] and to determine the persistence of *T. cruzi* in human tissues in the chronic stage of Chagas' disease.[64]

In a prenatal screening in Paraguay, from 7.7% to 10.5% of 2,000 pregnant women were serologically positive for *T. cruzi*.[65] Of 58 infants born to seropositive mothers, 2 were positive by direct microscopic observation at birth and 4 were PCR-positive but microscopy-negative at birth.

Differential Diagnosis With Other Species of Trypanosomatidae

Stained blood preparations allow differentiation of *T. cruzi* and *Trypanosoma rangeli*, whose ranges overlap in the north of South America and south of Central America.[1] In an endemic area for Chagas' disease in Venezuela, nine isolates of trypanosomes were identified as *T. rangeli* and 29.4% of the blood samples showed seropositivity for *T. cruzi*, an indication of the importance of coinfection with *T. cruzi* and *T. rangeli* in this region.[66] In addition, an anti-*T. rangeli* hyperimmune rabbit serum did not recognize the recombinant SAPA, which may allow a differential diagnosis in the acute phase of the Chagas' disease.[67] A variable domain from the large subunit ribosomal RNA gene has been used to amplify the total DNA of *T. rangeli* and *T. cruzi* and distinguish between species.[68] Species-specific detection of *T. cruzi* and *T. rangeli* in vector and mammalian hosts was done by PCR amplification of kinetoplast minicircle DNA. With S35/S36 primers in mice with single and mixed infections of *Rhodnius prolixus* and BALB/c, the profile of each trypanosome was easily distinguishable, in agreement with the localization of the parasite in the insect.[69] The mini-exon-derived probes for *T. cruzi*, *T. rangeli*, and *Trypanosoma brucei* were species-specific. This method, involving the detection of specific PCR-amplified products produced by a single primer set, represents a novel, sensitive, and specific assay for multiple trypanosomatid species and groups.[70]

Prognosis: Markers and Physiology of Chronic Chagas' Disease

Research on *T. cruzi* proteins that share the antigenic determinants of the host could reveal the self-aggressive autoimmune response or the ability of *T. cruzi* to take proteins from the medium and metabolize them, thus incorporating parasite peptides that may have the same epitopes as those in host tissues. Diagnostic techniques are being developed with recombinant proteins and antigens from the microsomal fraction of epimastigotes purified with monoclonal antibodies.[71,72] A DNA sequence of 188 bp of *T. cruzi* found in heart tissue of infected persons who also had cardiac inflammatory infiltrations and disease symptoms concordant with Chagas' disease has been revealed by PCR.[73] However, because this sequence was absent in the heart tissue of noninfected patients,[73] *T. cruzi* could be crucial in the pathogenesis of Chagas' disease.[74] These results are promising, but field trials must be carried out before these techniques can be recommended for patient orientation. In addition, the strong association between the occurrence of circulating myocardial antineurotransmitter receptor antibodies in patients with Chagas' disease and dysautonomic symptoms suggests that these antibodies are an early marker of autonomic dysfunction of the heart.[74]

Recombinant proteins of *T. cruzi* are also used for assessing treatment efficacy in acute and recent infections in children 6 to 12 years old. A mucin-like glycoconjugate anchored by glycocyl-phosphatidylinositol from cell-cultured trypomastigotes (AT) was used as antigen in a chemoluminescence assay, and a calcium binding protein (F29) was successfully used in an immunoenzymatic assay for the same purpose.[75,76] These reactions have also been tested in double-blind assays.

Markers for Follow-Up of Anti-*T. cruzi* Chemotherapy

The follow-up of patients treated with specific chemotherapy is accepted as a key for success. During the acute phase, treatment efficacy is easy to determine by the absence of parasitemia and reversion of signs and symptoms. In the indeterminate phase, however, neither easily detectable parasitemia nor signs or symptoms exist. In this phase, assessment of the progress of the patient relies on changes in the serodiagnosis or the appearance or disappearance of immune response markers.

Sera from patients chronically infected with *T. cruzi* display antibodies that bind to epitopes of live trypomastigotes, known as lytic antibodies, which are detected by a complement-mediated lysis test. Conventional serology antibodies are also present in sera from patients with chronic infections but, in contrast to lytic antibodies, are unable to recognize viable trypomastigotes. The presence of lytic antibodies has been considered a criterion of cure in human Chagas' disease. Sera from these patients were analyzed in a cytometer and antibodies identified on the basis of size and granularity gain adjustments. On the basis of experience with the complement-mediated lysis test, a level of 20% of parasites positive by fluorescein isothiocyanate fluorescence was used as a cutoff between effective and ineffective treatments.[77]

In a randomized, double-blind trial in a rural area of Brazil endemic for Chagas' disease, 130 schoolchildren seropositive for *T. cruzi* were treated with benznidazole (7.5 mg/kg daily for 60 days by mouth) or placebo. Treatment of early chronic *T. cruzi* infection was safe and 55.8% effective in producing negative seroconversion of specific antibodies.[78] In children 6 to 12 years of age who were treated with benznidazole at 5 to 7 mg/kg per day during 60 days and followed up for 48 months, specific treatment was effective in the indeterminate phase, as demonstrated by a significant decrease in serologic titers when total antigens were used.[76] When a recombinant antigen was used, negativization of serologic results reached approximately 65%, and xenodiagnosis was completely negative in placebo-treated patients.

New antigenic molecules of *T. cruzi* have been adapted for specific serodiagnosis in the past 2 years.[76,78] These molecules are used to assess the effectiveness of chemotherapy against *T. cruzi* infection, yielding important information for the physician. Diagnostic methods are essential to accomplish the objective of eliminating vector and blood-mediated transmission of *T. cruzi* in the southern cone countries by 2000. Other Central American and Mesoamerican countries are initiating a similar program. Different species of triatomine bugs and different sensitivity to the same antigenic preparation are some of the challenges for these initiatives. In the Southern Cone Initiative, Uruguay has been declared under surveillance and Chile has no more cases of acute Chagas' disease. In Argentina, a projection of current seroprevalence rates of *T. cruzi* suggests that there will be no infected child under the age of 4 by 2006. Even if no new instance of *T. cruzi* infection occurs in Argentina, more than 2 million patients will still need medical assistance in the next 20 years.

Acknowledgment: I deeply thank Drs. Ricardo Gürtler and Miriam Postan for helpful revision of this manuscript.

References

1. Control of Chagas Disease: Report of a WHO Expert Committee. WHO Technical Report Series 811. Geneva, WHO, 1991
2. Blanco SB, Gürtler RE, Segura EL: El control de la transmisión congénita de *Trypanosoma cruzi* en Argentina. Rev Medicina (Buenos Aires) 59 Suppl 1:138, 1999
3. Rosenbaum MB: Chagasic cardiomyopathy. Prog Cardiovasc Dis 7:199-225, 1964
4. Brener Z: Laboratory-acquired Chagas' disease an endemic disease among parasitology. The proceedings of the course of genes and antigens of Parasites. Edited by C Morel. Rio de Janeiro, 1984, p 883
5. Hoare CA: The Trypanosomes of Mammals: A Zoological Monograph. Oxford, Blackwell Scientific Publications, 1972, p 30
6. Zeledon R, Alvarenga NJ, Schosinsky K: Ecology of *Trypanosoma cruzi* in the Insect Vector. Washington, DC, PAHO Scientific Publications, 1977, p 347
7. Romaña C: Enfermedad de Chagas. Buenos Aires, López Libreros, 1963, p 42
8. Dvorak JA, Hyde TP: *Trypanosoma cruzi*: interaction with vertebrate cells in vitro. 1. Individual interactions at the cellular and subcellular levels. Exp Parasitol 34:268-283, 1973
9. Días JCP: História natural in Cardiopatía Chagásica. Edited by JR Cançado, M Chuster. Fundação Carlos Chagas, Belo Horizonte, 1985
10. Parada H, Carrasco HA, Anez N, Fuenmayor C, Inglessis I: Cardiac involvement is a constant finding in acute Chagas' disease: a clinical, parasitological and histopathological study. Int J Cardiol 60:49-54, 1997

11. Higuchi MD, Ries MM, Aiello VD, Benvenuti LA, Gutierrez PS, Bellotti G, Pileggi F: Association of an increase in CD8+ T cells with the presence of *Trypanosoma cruzi* antigens in chronic, human, chagasic myocarditis. Am J Trop Med Hyg 56:485-489, 1997

12. Petry K, Eisen H: Chagas disease: a model for the study of autoimmune diseases. Parasitol Today 5:111-116, 1989

13. Reis MM, Higuchi M de L, Benvenuti LA, Aiello VD, Gutierrez PS, Bellotti G, Pileggi F: An in situ quantitative immunohistochemical study of cytokines and IL-2R+ in chronic human chagasic myocarditis: correlation with the presence of myocardial *Trypanosoma cruzi* antigens. Clin Immunol Immunopathol 83:165-172, 1997

14. Viotti R, Vigliano C, Armenti H, Segura E: Treatment of chronic Chagas' disease with benznidazole: clinical and serologic evolution of patients with long-term follow-up. Am Heart J 127:151-162, 1994

15. Chuit R, Subias E, Perez AC, Paulone I, Wisnivesky-Colli C, Segura EL: Usefulness of serology for the evaluation of *Trypanosoma cruzi* transmission in endemic areas of Chagas' disease. Rev Soc Bras Med Trop 22:119-124, 1989

16. Cerisola JA, Rohweder R, Segura EL, del Prado CE, Alvarez M, Martini GJW: El xenodiagnóstico. Normatización, utilidad, Ministerio de Bienestar Social., Secret. de Estado de Salud Pública, Buenos Aires, 1974

17. Strout RG: A method for concentrating hemoflagellates. J Parasitol 48:100, 1962

18. Feilij H, Muller L, Gonzalez Cappa SM: Direct micromethod for diagnosis of acute and congenital Chagas' disease. J Clin Microbiol 18:327-330, 1983

19. Schenone H, Alfaro E, Reyes H, Taucher E: Value of xenodiagnosis in chronic Chagasic infection [Spanish]. Bol Chil Parasitol 23:149-154, 1968

20. Segura E: Xenodiagnosis. *In* Chagas' Disease Vectors. Edited by A de Stoka, R Brenner. Boca Raton, CRS Press, 1988, p 41

21. Pineda JP, Luquetti A, Castro C: Comparison between classical and artificial xenodiagnosis in chronic Chagas disease [Portuguese]. Rev Soc Bras Med Trop 31:473-480, 1998

22. Schenone H, Contreras MC, Rojas A, Villarroel F: Positivity of xenodiagnosis, according to age, in persons with positive serology for Chagas disease [Spanish]. Bol Chil Parasitol 50:42-44, 1995

23. Gürtler RE, Cecere MC, Castanera MB, Canale D, Lauricella MA, Chuit R, Cohen JE, Segura EL: Probability of infection with *Trypanosoma cruzi* of the vector Triatoma infestans fed on infected humans and dogs in northwest Argentina. Am J Trop Med Hyg 55:24-31, 1996

24. Wynne de Martini GJ, Abramo Orrego L, de Rissio AM, Alvarez M, Mujica LP: Culture of *Trypanosoma cruzi* in a monophasic medium. Application to large-scale cultures in fermentation processes [Spanish]. Medicina (B Aires) 40 Suppl 1:109-114, 1980

25. Chiari E, Días JC, Lana M, Chiari CA: Hemocultures for the parasitological diagnosis of human chronic Chagas' disease. Rev Soc Bras Med Trop 22:19-23, 1989

26. Abramo Orrego L, Lansetti JC, Bozzini JP, Wynne de Martini GJ: Hemoculture as a diagnostic method in Chagas disease [Spanish]. Medicina (B Aires) 40 Suppl 1:56-62, 1980

27. Galvao LMC, Cançado JR, Brener Z, Krettli AU: Hemoculture repeatedly negative in humans with Chagas' disease displaying negative complement-

mediated lysis tests after specific treatment suggest cure in infection. Mem Inst Oswaldo Cruz 81:111, 1981

28. Anez N, Carrasco H, Parada H, Crisante G, Rojas A, Gonzalez N, Ramirez JL, Guevara P, Rivero C, Borges R, Scorza JV: Acute Chagas' disease in western Venezuela: a clinical, seroparasitologic, and epidemiologic study. Am J Trop Med Hyg 60:215-222, 1999

29. Riarte A, Cantarovich M, Sinagra A, Alvarez A, del Prado C, Tizado J, Castro L, Segura EL: Reactivation of chronic Chagas disease and kidney transplant (abstract). J Protozool 38: , 1991

30. Cerisola JA: Serologic findings in patients with acute Chagas' disease treated with Bay 2502 [Spanish]. Bol Chil Parasitol 24:54-59, 1969

31. Cerisola JA: Chemotherapy of Chagas' infection in man. PAHO Scientific Publication 347, Washington, DC, PAHO, 1977

32. Zeledon R, Dias JC, Brilla-Salazar A, de Rezende JM, Vargas LG, Urbina A: Does a spontaneous cure for Chagas' disease exist? Rev Soc Bras Med Trop 21:15-20, 1988

33. Cura EN, Segura EL: Quality assurance of the serologic diagnosis of Chagas' disease. Rev Panam Salud Publica 3:242-248, 1998

34. Lauricella MA, Castanera MB, Gurtler RE, Segura EL: Immunodiagnosis of Trypanosoma cruzi (Chagas' disease) infection in naturally infected dogs. Mem Inst Oswaldo Cruz 93:501-507, 1998

35. Maekelt GA: Fracciones antigénicas del Schizotrypanum cruzi como fijador de complemento. Archivos Venezolanos de Medicina Tropical y Parasitologia Médica 4:213, 1962

36. Vattuone NH, Yanovsky JF: Trypanosoma cruzi: agglutination activity of enzyme-treated epimastigotes. Exp Parasitol 30:349-355, 1971

37. Rabello A, Luquetti AO, Moreira EF, Gadelha M de F, dos Santos JA, de Melo L, Schwind P: Serodiagnosis of Trypanosoma cruzi infection using the new particle gel immunoassay—ID-PaGIA Chagas. Mem Inst Oswaldo Cruz 94:77-82, 1999

38. Lansetti JC, Giordano AD, Subias E, Segura EL: Serologic screening tests for Chagas infection (letter) [Spanish]. Medicina (B Aires) 40 Suppl 1:258-259, 1980

39. Camargo ME, Hoshino S, Siqueira GR: Hemagglutination with preserved, sensitized cells, a practical test for routine serologic diagnosis of American trypanosomiasis. Rev Inst Med Trop Sao Paulo 15:81-85, 1973

40. Camargo ME, Segura EL, Kagan IG, Souza JM, Carvalheiro J da R, Yanovsky JF, Guimaraes MC: Three years of collaboration on the standardization of Chagas' disease serodiagnosis in the Americas: an appraisal. Bull Pan Am Health Organ 20:233-244, 1986

41. Salles NA, Sabino EC, Cliquet MG, Eluf-Neto J, Mayer A, Almeida-Neto C, Mendonca MC, Dorliach-Llacer P, Chamone DF, Saez-Alquezar A: Risk of exposure to Chagas' disease among seroreactive Brazilian blood donors. Transfusion 36:969-973, 1996

42. Alvarez M, Cerisola JA, Rohwedder RW: Immunofluorescence test in the diagnosis of Chagas' diseases [Spanish]. Bol Chil Parasitol 23:4-8, 1968

43. Camargo ME, Hoshino-Shimizu S: Metodologia sorológica na infeccao pelo Trypanosoma cruzi. Revista Goiania de Medicina 20:47, 1974

44. Camargo ME, Ferreira AW, Peres BA, Previato LM, Scharfstein J: Trypanosoma cruzi antibodies, in Bergmeyer. Methods of Enzymatic Analysis 11:368, 1986

45. Umezawa ES, Bastos SF, Camargo ME, Yamauchi LM, Santos MR, Gonzalez A, Zingales B, Levin MJ, Sousa O, Rangel-Aldao R, da Silveira JF: Evaluation of recombinant antigens for serodiagnosis of Chagas' disease in South and Central America. J Clin Microbiol 37:1554-1560, 1999

46. Houghton RL, Benson DR, Reynolds LD, McNeill PD, Sleath PR, Lodes MJ, Skeiky YA, Leiby DA, Badaro R, Reed SG: A multi-epitope synthetic peptide and recombinant protein for the detection of antibodies to *Trypanosoma cruzi* in radioimmunoprecipitation-confirmed and consensus-positive sera. J Infect Dis 179:1226-1234, 1999

47. Breniere SF, Yaksic N, Telleria J, Bosseno MF, Noireau F, Wincker P, Sanchez D: Immune response to *Trypanosoma cruzi* shed acute phase antigen in children from an endemic area for Chagas' disease in Bolivia. Mem Inst Oswaldo Cruz 92:503-507, 1997

48. Corral RS, Altcheh JM, Freilij HL: Presence of IgM antibodies to *Trypanosoma cruzi* urinary antigen in sera from patients with acute Chagas' disease. Int J Parasitol 28:589-594, 1998

49. Umezawa ES, Nascimento MS, Kesper N Jr, Coura JR, Borges-Pereira J, Junqueira AC, Camargo ME: Immunoblot assay using excreted-secreted antigens of *Trypanosoma cruzi* in serodiagnosis of congenital, acute, and chronic Chagas' disease. J Clin Microbiol 34:2143-2147, 1996

50. Morel C, Chiari E, Camargo EP, Mattei DM, Romanha AJ, Simpson L: Strains and clones of *Trypanosoma cruzi* can be characterized by pattern of restriction endonuclease products of kinetoplast DNA minicircles. Proc Natl Acad Sci U S A 77:6810-6814, 1980

51. Morel C, Deane M, Goncalves A: The complexity of *Trypanosoma cruzi* populations revealed by schizodeme analysis. Parasitology Today 2: , 1986

52. Frasch AC, Goijman SG, Cazzulo JJ, Stoppani AO: Constant and variable regions in DNA mini-circles from *Trypanosoma cruzi* and *Trypanosoma rangeli*: application to species and stock differentiation. Mol Biochem Parasitol 4:163-170, 1981

53. Tibayrenc M, Ward P, Moya A, Ayala FJ: Natural populations of *Trypanosoma cruzi*, the agent of Chagas disease, have a complex multiclonal structure. Proc Natl Acad Sci U S A 83:115-119, 1986

54. Degrave WM: Molecular diagnosis of Chagas disease. *In* Chagas Disease (American Trypanosomiasis): Its Impact on Transfusion and Clinical Medicine. Edited by S Wendel, Z Brener, ME Camargo, A Rassi. ISTB Brazil '92. Sao Paulo, Brazil 225, 1992

55. Moser DR, Kirchhoff LV, Donelson JE: Detection of *Trypanosoma cruzi* by DNA amplification using the polymerase chain reaction. J Clin Microbiol 27:1477-1482, 1989

56. Sturm NR, Degrave W, Morel C, Simpson L: Sensitive detection and schizodeme classification of *Trypanosoma cruzi* cells by amplification of kinetoplast minicircle DNA sequences: use in diagnosis of Chagas' disease. Mol Biochem Parasitol 33:205-214, 1989

57. Avila HA, Sigman DS, Cohen LM, Millikan RC, Simpson L: Polymerase chain reaction amplification of *Trypanosoma cruzi* kinetoplast minicircle DNA isolated from whole blood lysates: diagnosis of chronic Chagas' disease. Mol Biochem Parasitol 48:211-221, 1991

58. Gonzalez N, Galindo I, Guevara P, Novak E, Scorza JV, Anez N, Da Silveira JF, Ramirez JL: Identification and detection of *Trypanosoma cruzi* by using

a DNA amplification fingerprint obtained from the ribosomal intergenic spacer. J Clin Microbiol 32:153-158, 1994

59. Souto RP, Zingales B: Sensitive detection and strain classification of *Trypanosoma cruzi* by amplification of a ribosomal RNA sequence. Mol Biochem Parasitol 62:45-52, 1993

60. Silber AM, Bua J, Porcel BM, Segura EL, Ruiz AM: *Trypanosoma cruzi*: specific detection of parasites by PCR in infected humans and vectors using a set of primers (BP1/BP2) targeted to a nuclear DNA sequence. Exp Parasitol 85:225-232, 1997

61. Gomes ML, Galvao LM, Macedo AM, Pena SD, Chiari E: Chagas' disease diagnosis: comparative analysis of parasitologic, molecular, and serologic methods. Am J Trop Med Hyg 60:205-210, 1999

62. Gomes ML, Macedo AM, Vago AR, Pena SD, Galvao LM, Chiari E: *Trypanosoma cruzi*: optimization of polymerase chain reaction for detection in human blood. Exp Parasitol 88:28-33, 1998

63. Russomando G, Rojas de Arias A, Almiron M, Figueredo A, Ferreira ME, Morita K: *Trypanosoma cruzi*: polymerase chain reaction-based detection in dried feces of *Triatoma infestans*. Exp Parasitol 83:62-66, 1996

64. Anez N, Carrasco N, Parada H, Crisante G, Rojas A, Fuenmayor C, Gonzalez N, Percoco G, Borges R, Guevara P, Ramirez JL: Myocardial parasite persistence in chronic chagasic patients. Am J Trop Med Hyg 60:726-732, 1999

65. Russomando G, de Tomassone MM, de Guillen I, Acosta N, Vera N, Almiron M, Candia N, Calcena MF, Figueredo A: Treatment of congenital Chagas' disease diagnosed and followed up by the polymerase chain reaction. Am J Trop Med Hyg 59:487-491, 1998

66. Araque W, Plasencia E, Cortes C, Contreras V: Field evaluation of a diagnostic protocol for Chagas' disease and rangeliosis. Acta Cient Venez 47:238-243, 1996

67. Saldana A, Sousa OE, Orn A: Immunoparasitological studies of *Trypanosoma cruzi* low virulence clones from Panama: humoral immune responses and antigenic cross-reactions with *Trypanosoma rangeli* in experimentally infected mice. Scand J Immunol 42:644-650, 1995

68. Vallejo GA, Guhl F, Chiari E, Macedo AM: Species specific detection of *Trypanosoma cruzi* and *Trypanosoma rangeli* in vector and mammalian hosts by polymerase chain reaction amplification of kinetoplast minicircle DNA. Acta Trop 72:203-212, 1999

69. Ramos A, Maslov DA, Fernandes O, Campbell DA, Simpson L: Detection and identification of human pathogenic Leishmania and Trypanosoma species by hybridization of PCR-amplified mini-exon repeats. Exp Parasitol 82:242-250, 1996

70. Levin MJ, Mesri E, Benarous R, Levitus G, Schijman A, Levy-Yeyati P, Chiale PA, Ruiz AM, Kahn A, Rosenbaum MB, Torres HN, Segura EL: Identification of major *Trypanosoma cruzi* antigenic determinants in chronic Chagas' heart disease. Am J Trop Med Hyg 41:530-538, 1989

71. de Titto EH, Moreno M, Braun M, Segura EL: Chagas' disease: humoral response to subcellular fraction of *Trypanosoma cruzi* in symptomatic and asymptomatic patients. Trop Med Parasitol 38:163-166, 1987

72. Jones EM, Colley DG, Tostes S, Lopes ER, Vnencak-Jones CL, McCurley TL: Amplification of a *Trypanosoma cruzi* DNA sequence from inflamma-

tory lesions in human chagasic cardiomyopathy. Am J Trop Med Hyg 48:348-357, 1993

73. Borda ES, Sterin-Borda L: Antiadrenergic and muscarine receptor antibodies in Chagas' cardiomyopathy. Int J Cardiol 54:149-156, 1996

74. de Andrade AL, Zicker F, de Oliveira RM, Almeida Silva S, Luquetti A, Travassos LR, Almeida IC, de Andrade SS, de Andrade JG, Martelli CM: Randomised trial of efficacy of benznidazole in treatment of early *Trypanosoma cruzi* infection. Lancet 348:1407-1413, 1996

75. Sosa Estani S, Segura EL, Ruiz AM, Velazquez E, Porcel BM, Yampotis C: Efficacy of chemotherapy with benznidazole in children in the indeterminate phase of Chagas' disease. Am J Trop Med Hyg 59:526-529, 1998

76. Schmunis GA, Zicker F, Moncayo A: Interruption of Chagas' disease transmission through vector elimination (letter). Lancet 348:1171, 1996

77. Guevara AG, Taibi A, Alava J, Guderian RH, Ouaissi A: Use of a recombinant *Trypanosoma cruzi* protein antigen to monitor cure of Chagas disease. Trans R Soc Trop Med Hyg 89:447-448, 1995

78. Esquivel ML, Segura EL: Calculating the number of patients with Chagas disease in Argentina (letter) [Spanish]. Medicina (B Aires) 54:91-92, 1994

Chapter 3

Molecular Pathology of Chagas' Disease

Mariano J. Levin, M.D.

With the advent of molecular biology, molecular genetics, and genomics, novel insights on the pathogenic mechanisms underlying chronic Chagas' heart disease have been obtained.

Cloned Parasite Antigens Allow Differentiation of the Acute From the Chronic Phase of the Disease

One of the most interesting findings, often overlooked, directly associated with the cloning of *Trypanosoma cruzi* antigens is that the acute and chronic phases of the disease are characterized by distinct, clearly different antibody profiles.[1] Whereas 90% of patients with acute Chagas' disease have antibodies to a membrane-anchored, trypomastigote-specific protein (shed acute phase antigen [SAPA]), only 10% of patients with chronic disease have anti-SAPA antibodies.[2] On the other hand, 90% to 100% of the patients with chronic disease have IgG antibodies against intracellular parasite proteins,[1,3] whereas these are detected in only 20% to 40% of sera from patients in the acute phase. These results may be summarized as follows: (1) Each phase of the disease can be distinguished not only by specific clinical symptoms but also by a specific set of anti-*T. cruzi* antibodies, and (2) the antibody patterns detected by cloned parasite antigens may be used in the differential diagnosis of the acute and chronic phases of the infection.[1,3]

Another possibility derived from these results and from additional data presented by Masuda et al.[4] is that in the acute phase, the main targets of the humoral response are parasite surface or secreted mole-

From Tentori MC, Segura EL, Hayes DL (eds.) *Arrhythmia Management in Chagas' Disease.* Armonk, NY: Futura Publishing Co., Inc. ©2000.

19

cules, implying undestroyed parasite cells because circulating parasites are detected, whereas in the chronic phase, the predominant targets of the immune system are intracellular proteins, suggesting an active rupture of parasite cells at this phase of the disease. Most interestingly, antibodies elicited against typical intracellular proteins, such as the ribosomal P proteins, have a functional effect on heart cells and tissue (see below).

High Levels of Antibodies Against Parasite Intracellular Proteins Are Associated With Foci of Myocarditis or Severe Chagas' Heart Disease

Within the past few years, my group has described the antibody response against the ribosomal P proteins in chronic Chagas' heart disease (cChHD). The main epitopes of the two types of ribosomal P proteins are located in the C-terminal ends of the low-molecular-weight ribosomal P1 and P2 proteins (peptide R13, EEEDDDMGFGLFD)[3,5] and of the P0-38 kd polypeptide (peptide P0-18, including peptide P0-β).[6,7] High antibody responses against peptide R13 have been detected in patients with cChHD.[3,5,8] Further studies established an association between myocarditis and anti-R13 antibody levels. Sera from patients with cChHD and histologic evidence of myocarditis show significantly higher anti-R13 levels than those measured in patients with cChHD without myocarditis.[9-11]

Particularly relevant to this brief description is the case of reference patient JL.[3,12] The serum of patient JL was used as an immunologic probe for isolating parasite recombinant antigens from a *T. cruzi* expression library.[3] Patient JL died with congestive heart failure at age 27; he was in New York Heart Association functional class IV. His electrocardiogram at admission in 1985, at age 25, showed first-degree atrioventricular block, left anterior fascicular block, and an area of anterior electrical inactivation. After 1 year of follow-up, he had right bundle branch block, premature ventricular contractions (Lown 4), and complete atrioventricular block.[12] A strong anti-R13 response was detected in the serum of patient JL,[3,5] implying that he had broken parasite cells somewhere in his system and that these high antibody levels were associated with foci of myocardial inflammation. Microscopic analysis of heart tissue samples at necropsy confirmed myocarditis but did not show signs of parasite nests or cells. However, polymerase chain reaction analysis of paraffin-embedded heart muscle samples allowed amplification of a 330-bp *T. cruzi* minicircle DNA fragment, pointing to the existence of the parasite in this organ.[12] Detection of *T. cruzi* DNA in heart tissue suggests that heart parasitization is a prevalent stimulus for the perpetuation of myocardial inflammation and for the generation of a strong humoral response, with high serum concentrations of antibodies against intracellular proteins and epitopes, such as R13.

Since parasite cells are so rare, or even nonapparent in sites of myocardial inflammation, detection of parasite DNA or parasite antigens and strong humoral responses against intracellular components associated with inflammatory foci imply an active and efficient in situ breakdown of parasite cells. Further studies along this line of research may disclose mechanisms involved in a heart-specific response to infection.[13-15]

Analysis of the antibody response to other types of intracellular antigens, such as the flagellar antigen with repetitive motifs, namely, JL7, allowed Kaplan et al.[16] to postulate that antibody levels against JL7 are increased in patients with the most severe forms of cChHD.

Autoimmunity in Chagas' Disease: A Bystander Effect of the Strong Antiparasite Response

Several authors have described the existence of an autoimmune response in patients with cChHD (for a complete review of this matter, see the article by Kierszenbaum[17]). Cunha-Neto et al.[18] have been highly quoted for their description of a typical Chagas' disease autoantibody. The authors report the existence of a cardiac myosin-specific epitope, AAALDK, that would be able to support an antiheart response even without the parasite.[18] However, my collaborators and I have been completely unable to detect antibodies against AAALDK in patients with cChHD. Moreover, we could not confirm that the peptide AAALDK inhibited the binding of cChHD sera to a suggested cross-reactive parasite protein, B13.[17,19]

On the contrary, antibodies against parasite proteins may have the ability to react with their own proteins. This is the situation in which antibodies react with the R13 epitope, also known as anti-P antibodies, previously discussed. These antibodies recognize the peptide EEEDDDMGFGLFD, which shares homology with (1) the C-terminal region of the human ribosomal P proteins H13 and EESDDDMGFGLFD, in turn the target of anti-P autoantibodies in systemic lupus erythematosus (SLE), and (2) the acidic extracellular epitope of the β_1-adrenergic receptor AESDE.[7]

Anti-P antibodies from chagasic patients showed a marked preference for recombinant parasite ribosomal P proteins and peptides, whereas anti-P autoantibodies from SLE reacted with human and parasite ribosomal P proteins and peptides to the same extent. A semiquantitative estimation of the binding of cChHD anti-P antibodies to R13 and H13 with the use of biosensor technology indicated that the average affinity constant was about five times higher for R13 than for H13. Competitive immunoenzyme assays demonstrated that cChHD anti-P antibodies bind to the acidic portions of peptide H13 and to peptide H26R, encompassing the second extracellular loop of the β_1-adrenoceptor. Anti-P antibodies isolated from patients with cChHD exert a positive chronotropic effect in vitro on cardiomyocytes from neonatal rats, an effect closely resembling that of anti-β_1-receptor antibodies isolated from the same patient. In contrast, SLE anti-P autoantibodies have no functional effect.[8] The results suggest that the adrenergic-stimulating activity of anti-P antibodies may be at the origin of functional impairments occurring in cChHD, a hypothesis reinforced by the finding that immunization with the ribosomal P2-β protein induces electrocardiographic changes in immunized mice[20] and by data presented by Masuda et al.[4] from work on isolated rabbit hearts.

Study of the properties of the anti-P antibodies in Chagas' disease shows clearly that the antibodies generated in this chronic infection are directed against the parasite and are not systemic autoantibodies. This conclusion dismisses the involvement of systemic autoimmune mechanisms in the generation of chagasic disease.

The *T. cruzi* Genome Project: An Efficient Way to Study the Parasite

T. cruzi is central in the establishment of the chronic infection and its clinical consequences. Thus, understanding of the molecular basis of parasite behavior seems urgently needed. The *T. cruzi* genome project is quickly providing a massive input of information. The repertoire of expressed genes (7,200 ESTs) is growing steadily, and chromosomal sequences of long stretches of DNA are now available. A first survey of the results of the project indicates that the genome of the parasite shows evidence of a dynamic conformation. Results from laboratories associated with this initiative have characterized genes and genomic regions that show chromatid rearrangements, movements of genes to telomeric regions, and novel virulence factors[21-23] pointing to a highly flexible and probably highly interactive genome. In all cases, a repetitive nuclear sequence that my collaborators and I have named "SIRE" seems to be involved.[24]

This approach to genomics has prompted us to try to detect and sequence fragments of the parasite genome at the site of the cardiac lesion (cardiac biopsies) in an attempt to analyze parasites directly linked to inflammation. This has been accomplished by micromanipulation techniques.[25] The results of the amplification and ulterior sequence of the amplified fragments showed great conservation of the amplicons of SIRE, a nuclear sequence, but great variability in sequence of the amplicons derived from the variable region of the minicircle. These results are only the first steps of an analysis that should lead us to understanding the active human-infecting parasite.[25] In turn, the human genome project will provide elements to complete the analysis of the genetic background of individuals, families, and populations most affected by the cardiac form of this chronic disease.

Novel research projects such as those discussed should pave the way to a more complete understanding of Chagas' disease and of its most severe expression, cChHD. They should further lead to design protocols to neutralize the bystander effects of antiparasite antibodies, such as the anti-P, and to development of more efficient and reliable antiparasitic therapies.

Acknowledgments: Work reported in this review was supported by grants of UNDP/ World Bank/WHO Special Programme for Research and Training in Tropical Diseases; European Commission contract 936018 AR; Programa Iberoamericano de Ciencia y Tecnología para el Desarrollo (CYTED); University of Buenos Aires; *T. cruzi* genome project of CABBIO (1996-1998); CONICET and FONCyT BID 802/OC-AR PICT 01421 y PICT 02030. M.J.L. is John Simon Guggenheim Memorial Foundation Fellow (1998-1999).

References

1. Levin MJ, Franco da Silveira J, Frasch AC, Camargo ME, Lavon S, Degrave WM, Rangel-Aldao R: Recombinant *Trypanosoma cruzi* antigens and Chagas' disease diagnosis: analysis of a workshop. FEMS Microbiol Immunol 4:11-19, 1991
2. Affranchino JL, Ibanez CF, Luquetti AO, Rassi A, Reyes MB, Macina RA, Aslund L, Pettersson U, Frasch AC: Identification of a *Trypanosoma cruzi* antigen that is shed during the acute phase of Chagas' disease. Mol Biochem Parasitol 34:221-228, 1989
3. Levin MJ, Mesri E, Benarous R, Levitus G, Schijman A, Levy-Yeyati P, Chiale PA, Ruiz AM, Kahn A, Rosenbaum MB, Torres HN, Segura EL: Identification of major *Trypanosoma cruzi* antigenic determinants in chronic Chagas' heart disease. Am J Trop Med Hyg 41:530-538, 1989
4. Masuda MO, Levin M, De Oliveira SF, Dos Santos Costa PC, Bergami PL, Dos Santos Almeida NA, Pedrosa RC, Ferrari I, Hoebeke J, Campos de Carvalho AC: Functionally active cardiac antibodies in chronic Chagas' disease are specifically blocked by *Trypanosoma cruzi* antigens. FASEB J 12:1551-1558, 1998
5. Levin MJ, Vazquez M, Kaplan D, Schijman AG: The *Trypanosoma cruzi* ribosomal P protein family: classification and antigenicity. Parasitol Today 9:381-384, 1993
6. Schijman AG, Levitus G, Levin MJ: Characterization of the C-terminal region of a *Trypanosoma cruzi* 38-kDa ribosomal P0 protein that does not react with lupus anti-P autoantibodies. Immunol Lett 33:15-20, 1992
7. Ferrari I, Levin MJ, Wallukat G, Elies R, Lebesgue D, Chiale P, Elizari M, Rosenbaum M, Hoebeke J: Molecular mimicry between the immunodominant ribosomal protein P0 of *Trypanosoma cruzi* and a functional epitope on the human beta 1-adrenergic receptor. J Exp Med 182:59-65, 1995
8. Kaplan D, Ferrari I, Bergami PL, Mahler E, Levitus G, Chiale P, Hoebeke J, Van Regenmortel MH, Levin MJ: Antibodies to ribosomal P proteins of *Trypanosoma cruzi* in Chagas disease possess functional autoreactivity

with heart tissue and differ from anti-P autoantibodies in lupus. Proc Natl Acad Sci U S A 94:10301-10306, 1997

9. Levin MJ: Molecular mimicry and Chagas' heart disease: high anti-R-13 autoantibody levels are markers of severe Chagas heart complaint. Res Immunol 142:157-159, 1991

10. Levin MJ, Kaplan D, Ferrari I, Arteman P, Vazquez M, Panebra A: Humoral autoimmune response in Chagas' disease: *Trypanosoma cruzi* ribosomal antigens as immunizing agents. FEMS Immunol Med Microbiol 7:205-210, 1993

11. Aznar C, Lopez-Bergami P, Brandariz S, Mariette C, Liegeard P, Alves MD, Barreiro EL, Carrasco R, Lafon S, Kaplan D, et al: Prevalence of anti-R-13 antibodies in human *Trypanosoma cruzi* infection. FEMS Immunol Med Microbiol 12:231-238, 1995

12. Brandariz S, Schijman A, Vigliano C, Arteman P, Viotti R, Beldjord C, Levin MJ: Detection of parasite DNA in Chagas' heart disease (letter). Lancet 346:1370-1371, 1995

13. Bestetti RB: Role of parasites in the pathogenesis of Chagas' cardiomyopathy (letter). Lancet 347:913-914, 1996

14. Levin MJ: In chronic Chagas heart disease, don't forget the parasite. Parasitol Today 12:415-416, 1996

15. Levin MJ: More on Chagas' disease cardiomyopathy. Parasitol Today 13:362-363, 1997

16. Kaplan D, Brandariz S, Degrave W, Desouza L, Luquetti A, Lopez Bergami P, Arteman P, Levin MJ: A new recombinant reactive reagent for Chagas' disease ELISA diagnosis. Mem Inst Oswaldo Cruz 90 Suppl 1:178, 1995

17. Kierszenbaum F: Chagas' disease and the autoimmunity hypothesis. Clin Microbiol Rev 12:210-223, 1999

18. Cunha-Neto E, Duranti M, Gruber A, Zingales B, De Messias I, Stolf N, Bellotti G, Patarroyo ME, Pilleggi F, Kalil J: Autoimmunity in Chagas' disease cardiopathy: biological relevance of a cardiac myosin-specific epitope crossreactive to an immunodominant *Trypanosoma cruzi* antigen. Proc Natl Acad Sci U S A 92:3541-3545, 1995

19. Ferrari I, Kaplan D, Mahler E, López Bergami P, Quintana F, Ghio S, Levitus G, Levin MJ: Generation of antibodies with functional autoreactive properties in Chagas' disease. Mem Inst Oswaldo Cruz 93 Suppl 1:83-84, 1998

20. Lopez Bergami P, Cabeza Meckert P, Kaplan D, Levitus G, Elias F, Quintana F, Van Regenmortel M, Laguens R, Levin MJ: Immunization with recombinant *Trypanosoma cruzi* ribosomal P2beta protein induces changes in the electrocardiogram of immunized mice. FEMS Immunol Med Microbiol 18:75-85, 1997

21. Andersson B, Aslund L, Tammi M, Tran AN, Hoheisel JD, Pettersson U: Complete sequence of a 93.4-kb contig from chromosome 3 of *Trypanosoma cruzi* containing a strand-switch region. Genome Res 8:809-816, 1998

22. Chiurillo MA, Cano I, Da Silveira JF, Ramirez JL: Organization of telomeric and sub-telomeric regions of chromosomes from the protozoan parasite *Trypanosoma cruzi*. Mol Biochem Parasitol 100:173-183, 1999

23. Weston D, Patel B, Van Voorhis WC: Virulence in *Trypanosoma cruzi* infection correlates with the expression of a distinct family of sialidase superfamily genes. Mol Biochem Parasitol 98:105-116, 1999

24. Vázquez M, Lorenzi H, Schijman A, Ben-Dov C, Levin MJ: Analysis of the distribution of SIRE in the nuclear genome of *Trypanosoma cruzi* reveals its linkage to other repetitive sequences and protein coding genes. Gene (in press)
25. Ghío S, Elías F, López Bergami P, Lorenzi H, Mahler E, Ben-Dov C, Burgos J, Quintana F, Volchof R, Vázquez M, Schijman A, Levitus G, Berek C, González A, Levin MJ: Aportes del Proyecto Genoma de *Trypanosoma cruzi* a la comprensión de la patogénesis de la cardiomiopatía chagásica crónica. Medicina (B Aires) (in press)

Chapter 4

Clinical Aspects of Chagas' Disease

Juan José Puigbó, M.D., F.A.C.C.,
Harry Acquatella, M.D., F.A.C.C.,
Claudia Suárez, M.D.,
José Gregorio Loyo, M.D.,
Hugo Giordano, M.D.

Chagas' disease, or American trypanosomiasis, is a disease caused by the protozoan parasite *Trypanosoma cruzi*, affecting primarily, but not exclusively, the heart. In the advanced phase, this disease causes a chronic dilated cardiomyopathy. The disease is present only on the American continent, from northern Mexico to southern Argentina. Nearly 20 million people are estimated to be infected with the parasite, and about 100 million are at risk of becoming infected. In countries where the disease is found, it causes significant public health problems. In addition, an estimated one-half million infected persons are living in the United States as a result of migrations from other countries.[1]

Natural History

Chagas' disease evolves in three phases: acute, indeterminate, and chronic. Many variations of this classic pattern of evolution exist; for example, the acute phase may not have clinical manifestations, the intermediate phase may not advance, and the chronic phase may remain stable indefinitely.

From Tentori MC, Segura EL, Hayes DL (eds.) *Arrhythmia Management in Chagas' Disease.* Armonk, NY: Futura Publishing Co., Inc. ©2000.

Epidemiology

The etiologic agent, *T. cruzi*, is a hemoflagellate protozoan transmitted by an insect, a bloodsucking vector of the family Reduviidae, subfamily Triatominae. The most important vectors epidemiologically are *Triatoma infestans*, *Panstrongylus megistus* in southern countries, and *Rhodnius prolixus* in northern South America. Most transmission is from animal host to man by means of a reduviid that discharges the feces while sucking human blood. The bug's feces carry the *T. cruzi* that penetrates the body through the skin or mucous membranes.

Other mechanisms of transmission are blood transfusions from infected donors (serologic screening should be compulsory); transplacental spread, causing infection of the fetus or congenital Chagas' disease; transplantation of organs from infected donors; and means such as accidental contamination in laboratories, digestion, lactation, and sexual transmission.[2]

Pathogenesis

The mechanisms by which *T. cruzi* causes tissue damage have been the subject of many studies, but little is known. A histopathologic feature common to the acute and chronic phases is an inflammatory infiltrate. Although tissular parasitism is considerably reduced in the chronic phase, it is now thought that the parasite or its antigens are almost always present in the tissues.[3,4] The pathogenetic mechanisms that have been studied the most are direct action by the parasite, immunologically mediated tissue damage, microcirculation abnormalities, autonomic dysfunction, and abnormalities of the extracellular matrix[5] (see respective chapters).

Acute Chagas' Disease

General Comments

The most important manifestation is an acute myocarditis recognized by the constant presence of *T. cruzi* in peripheral blood. The clinically apparent form is characterized by a febrile illness accompanied by localized, systemic, and organic involvement. This florid form is the least frequent, whereas the asymptomatic and inapparent forms are the most frequent (95%). In areas of endemic disease, the manifestations may be a febrile illness of undetermined origin confirmed by parasitemia. Most acute cases occur during the first 2 years of life (85% of the cases), although acute Chagas' disease may appear at any age. The incubation period ranges from 1 to 2 weeks up to 1 month.

Local Manifestations

Romaña's eye sign, or ophthalmolymphangitis complex, is the most characteristic manifestation and is caused by *T. cruzi* transconjunctival penetration. This sign consists of elastic, nonpainful periocular and facial edema, almost always unilateral, with purplish erythema; conjunctivitis; and regional adenopathy with virtually no pain. It evolves in 1 to 2 months. Prevalence is extremely variable, depending on the geographical area and the degree of epidemiologic control.

Skin lesions include Mazza's inoculation chagoma, an initial inflammatory lesion found at the point of entry through the skin. The clinical aspect may vary from nodule to erythematous, furunculoid, or erysipelatoid plaque with regional adenopathy. Hematogenous or secondary chagomas can also occur. The genal lipochagoma affects the corpus adiposum buccae. It is generally found in nursing infants during the first year of life and is an extremely characteristic, but not very frequent, sign.

Systemic Manifestations

The systemic manifestations include a variable and nonspecific febrile syndrome, exanthemas, hepatosplenomegaly, lymphadenopathy, and anasarca.

Acute Chagas' Heart Disease

Involvement of the myocardium is constant during this phase, as shown by endomyocardial biopsy or autopsy,[6] but the severity of the involvement varies. In most cases (90% to 95%), the clinical course of the disease is benign, leading to death in only a minority (5% to 10%) of the patients. Severity is related to myocardial involvement (acute myocarditis) or neurologic involvement (meningoencephalitis). A change in prognosis is now possible with antiparasitic drug therapy.

Pathologic findings show florid acute myocarditis with the typical myocardial parasitism (amastigote forms). The frequency of histopathologic involvement of the myocardium is probably higher than has been clinically estimated.

The clinical manifestations of acute Chagas' myocarditis are nonspecific, except for the findings of *T. cruzi* in the peripheral blood. In some cases, cardiovascular test results may be normal, showing slight and nonspecific changes in the electrocardiogram (ECG). In patients with moderately severe symptoms, the most frequent finding is persistent and significant sinus tachycardia that is out of proportion to the fever. Arterial hypotension and functional heart murmurs may be found during the physical examination.

Radiographs show slight to moderate enlargement of the cardiovascular silhouette (in nearly 60%), with frequent pericardial effusion (Fig. 4-1 and 4-2).

ECGs show abnormalities in nearly 50% of the patients. Most of the findings, however, are nonspecific, such as ventricular repolarization disorders, first-degree atrioventricular block, and low voltage. These abnormalities are related to pancarditis and, especially, pericarditis and acute myocarditis. In general, the abnormalities tend to disappear and the ECG becomes normal. Infrequent findings of right bundle branch block and second-degree atrioventricular block during this phase have been mentioned as indicative of an ominous prognosis.[6] In severe forms (about 10%), the clinical examination shows cardiomegaly, significant enlargement of the cardiovascular silhouette in radiographs, massive pericardial effusion in the echocardiogram, and signs of ventricular dysfunction that may lead to death.

Echocardiography is extremely useful in studying Chagas' disease in general and, especially, in the acute phase. Echocardiograms dis-

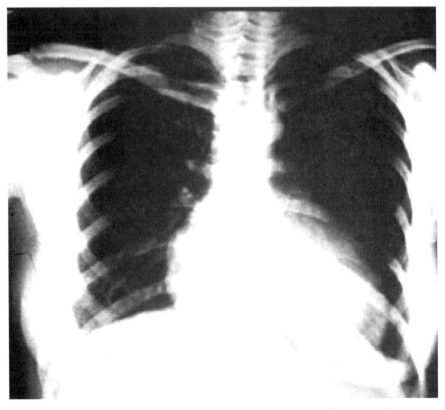

Fig. 4-1. Acute Chagas' disease. A 32-year-old woman had exertional dyspnea and fatigability, Romaña's sign on the right eye, and cardiomegaly by chest radiography. A normal ejection fraction of 55% was found.

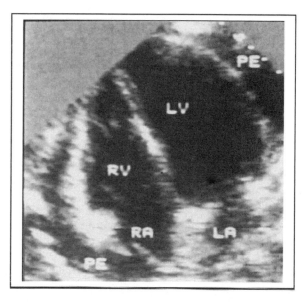

Fig. 4-2. Two-dimensional echocardiogram (same patient as in Fig. 4-1). Normal left ventricle (LV) size and ejection fraction. A large pericardial effusion (PE) is present. LA, left atrium; RA, right atrium; RV, right ventricle.

closed abnormalities in 52% of the patients studied (27 of 52) in a recent outbreak of acute Chagas' disease. The most significant findings[6] were as follows:

1. Frequent pericardial effusion (see Fig. 4-2) (42% of patients). Effusion was mild to moderate in 17 patients and severe in 5. Slight to moderate pericardial effusion was found even in patients without congestive heart failure.
2. Normal left ventricular ejection fraction in all patients studied. Right ventricular size was also normal. Anterior or apical dyskinesis of the left ventricle was found in 11 patients (21%) and left ventricular dilatation in 3 (6%). Four patients with heart failure died before being tested.

The principal finding in the 26 patients in the series[6] who had endomyocardial biopsy was acute, diffuse myocarditis with mononuclear and neutrophil inflammatory infiltrate associated with myofibrillar lesions. On the basis of the Dallas criteria, myocarditis was found without fibrosis in 16 biopsy specimens and with little fibrosis in 13. Endomyocardial biopsies repeated on an average of 8 years later in 14 patients showed evolving myocarditis with scarce fibrosis. The most characteristic but infrequent (2 of 26) finding was intracellular *T. cruzi* (nests of amastigotes). In postmortem studies, tissular parasitism is always present.

Neurologic Involvement

Neurologic disease consists of light to severe meningoencephalitis. In earlier days, the prognosis was unfavorable, with high mortality, especially in children younger than 2 years. At present, however, early diagnosis and etiologic treatment have led to better prognoses.

Laboratory Diagnosis

Diagnosis is by findings of *T. cruzi* in the circulating blood, by blood cultures, and by xenodiagnosis (specificity, 100%). Serologic test findings become positive, on the average, 1 month later. Testing of the cerebrospinal fluid is essential in patients with neurologic involvement.

Specific Treatment

Two antiparasitic drugs have been used, nifurtimox (a nitrofuran) and benznidazole (a nitroimidazole). The general criterion for considering that treatment has been successful is that both parasitemia and serologic test results become negative. In the series[6] mentioned above, the parasitemia findings were negative, but serologic test results were negative in only eight (20%) of the patients treated and the evolution of the myocarditis was not halted. Further studies on the efficacy of chemotherapy in Chagas' disease, especially over the long term, are needed.

Indeterminate Phase of Chagas' Disease

General Comments

The indeterminate phase follows cessation of the clinical manifestations in the apparent forms of acute Chagas' disease, with a reduction or apparent cessation of parasitemia. Most frequently, the patient has no history of acute Chagas' disease, is both seropositive and asymptomatic, and does not have objective evidence of heart or digestive disease. In addition, the pathologic substratum of this phase shows scarce tissue parasitism and mild morphologic abnormalities (mild myocarditis and fibrosis). This phase may last decades, but the precise duration is difficult to determine, both at the onset (the acute phase may not be apparent) and at the end (undefined onset of the chronic phase).

Differences in Evolution

In most patients (nearly 80%), this phase of the disease continues to the end of life, whereas in a minority (nearly 20%), it evolves to the chronic phase. In the vast majority of the latter patients, this evolution is gradual and without symptoms. It has been suggested that differences between the two groups are due to differences in the immunologic response. On the basis of autopsies of persons dying accidentally and of findings from endomyocardial biopsies, the indeterminate phase may represent a continuum from the acute to the chronic phase, with potentially different evolutionary patterns.

Pathologic Findings

Macroscopic findings[7] are productive epicarditis and, occasionally, the characteristic lesion of left ventricular apex thinning. Microscopic studies reveal slight focal myocarditis and fibrosis, perivasculitis, periganglionitis, and lesions in the conduction system.

Basis for the Diagnosis

The characteristics of the disease in this phase are

1. Antibodies to *T. cruzi* on serologic testing.
2. Low-grade parasitemia, usually difficult to detect (<20%).
3. Patients younger than 40 (20 to 40 years; average, 30 years), depending on whether a prophylactic program is in effect; prognosis is excellent, and the mortality rate is about the same as that for the general population.
4. No heart disease found in clinical examinations or by usual diagnostic methods.
5. No disease of the gastrointestinal system, especially of the esophagus (megaesophagus) or the colon (megacolon), which is found only in some areas of endemic Chagas' disease.

Evolution to the Chronic Phase

The crucial diagnostic issue is whether the disease is at the indeterminate phase without organ involvement or has evolved to the chronic phase of established heart disease.

Diagnostic Studies

ECG has proven to be a simple, low-cost procedure that, together with serologic tests, has been extremely useful in epidemiologic field studies. Diagnostic study results may be within normal limits or show early signs of chronic Chagas' heart disease:

1. Early segmental wall motion abnormalities and, occasionally, apical aneurysms are revealed by one or more of the following procedures: radionuclide angiography, echocardiography, and cardiac catheterization.
2. Abnormalities of the diastolic properties can also be detected by the second and third methods.
3. In approximately one-third of the patients, a treadmill stress test may show an arrhythmogenic tendency and a chronotropic deficit; the transition from a normal to an abnormal ECG usually reveals intraventricular conduction disorders.
4. In 60% of the patients, an endomyocardial biopsy may show an inflammatory process and, less frequently, fibrosis.
5. In certain areas of endemic disease, a gastrointestinal study may show evidence of megaesophagus or megacolon, which necessitates a cardiovascular evaluation to determine whether the abnormality is associated with heart disease.

Chronic Chagas' Disease

Chronic Chagas' cardiomyopathy is the main clinical and pathologic expression of Chagas' disease. This type of cardiomyopathy appears gradually as a nondilated cardiomyopathy with few clinical manifestations and progresses very slowly to a dilated cardiomyopathy principally manifested by arrhythmias, left ventricular dysfunction, embolic episodes, and autonomic dysfunction. Very specific and distinctive characteristics are early segmental wall motion abnormalities and an apical aneurysm. In general, the cause of death is sudden death, heart failure, or thromboembolic phenomena. Pathologically, Chagas' disease is one of the most frequent causes of chronic myocarditis. Myocardial lesions are progressive, self-perpetuating, and cumulative. The apical aneurysm is found to be a distinctive pathologic marker of this type of cardiomyopathy in more than 50% of patients with symptoms.

Natural History

Epidemiologic studies have made it possible to determine the natural history and, especially in the early stages before symptoms, to identify geographical differences in the disease and provide a basis for prevention. These studies have also shown that prevention programs (changes in rural housing and efforts to eradicate the vector with the use of insecticides) could bring about changes in the pattern of evolution of the disease (reduction or suppression of the acute phase and delay in onset of the chronic phase). According to a number of follow-up studies, heart disease develops in 20% to 30% of the patients with indeterminate-phase Chagas' disease one to several decades after infection, at a rate between 2% and 5% per year. In general, heart disease appears during the second or third decade of life. Heart failure generally occurs later, after the fourth decade, in endemic areas with no prevention programs and even later in areas with prevention programs. The death rate is 20% among patients in the 20- to 50-year-old range and is higher among men.

Pathologic Findings

The pathologic substrata of Chagas' heart disease are chronic, diffuse, evolving myocarditis with a tendency toward pronounced fibrosis and a characteristic marker, namely, an apical lesion or ventricular aneurysm of the apex, with its pronounced tendency to intracavity thrombosis (Fig. 4-3). In the early stages, the cardiomyopathy is nondilated, or type I (concentric), with ventricular hypertrophy, normal-sized left ventricular cavity, and a "closed" (circumscribed) apical lesion of the left ventricle (Fig. 4-3, panel A). This pattern is found after accidental or sudden death[7] with no evidence of heart failure. In advanced stages, or type II (eccentric) cardiomyopathy, predominant dilation of the left ventricular cavity, with an "open" (extended) apical lesion and frequent intracavity thrombosis (Fig. 4-3, panel C), is generally accompanied by global dilatation of the rest of the cavities. The characteristic apical lesion or aneurysm of the apex was found in 60% of our series and the posterior basal lesion in 20%. Histologically, the specific sign of parasitism of the fiber (nests of amastigotes) is found in 20% to 30% of the patients (Fig. 4-4).

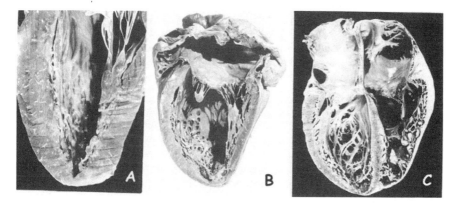

Fig. 4-3. Panel A: Chronic Chagas' disease, pathologic type I: left ventricular hypertrophy. Panel B: Intermediate type, showing apical thinning. Panel C: Dilatation of the left ventricle, apical thinning, and thrombosis.

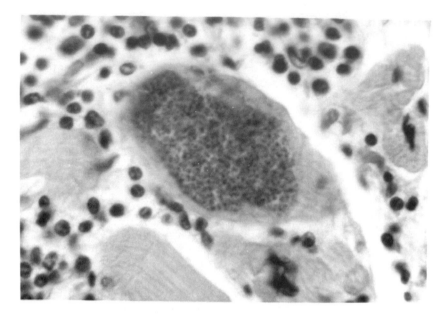

Fig. 4-4. Photomicrograph of ventricular myocardium in chronic Chagas' disease. An amastigote nest, as shown, may be found in 20% to 30% of patients with chronic disease.

Basis for the Diagnosis

In general, diagnoses of chronic Chagas' cardiomyopathy are based on the following characteristics:

1. *Positive epidemiologic data.* The patient's country and place of birth; residence in or arrival from an area where Chagas' disease is known to be endemic; type of dwelling; the patient's possible knowledge of the insect that bites and transmits the disease; blood transfusion from a carrier of the infection; the child of a mother with Chagas' disease.
2. *Blood tests positive for T. cruzi.* Several different tests are used: enzyme-linked immunosorbent assay, radioimmunoassay, indirect immunofluorescence, indirect hemagglutination, complement fixation test, and hemagglutination reaction. Positive results of at least two serologic tests are required.
3. *Diagnosis of cardiomyopathy.* Cardiomegaly, abnormal ECG (right bundle branch block, left anterior hemiblock, ventricular arrhythmia), areas of dyskinesis, or apical aneurysm.
4. *Absence of other types of heart disease.* Nevertheless, at 50 years of age or more, combined forms with hypertensive or ischemic heart disease may pose diagnostic difficulties.

Classification

Stratification and Grading

A sui generis characteristic of Chagas' disease is that it can be detected by serologic testing during the long-lasting (decades) asymptomatic stage, both in the indeterminate phase and in the early chronic phase. The New York Heart Association (NYHA) classification is extremely useful during the symptomatic stage, which appears late and is indicative of important risk factors for predicting mortality. Among diagnostic techniques that have been useful, echocardiography stands out as an extremely simple and valuable tool. The evolution of chronic Chagas' disease can be described and classified in three stages: early (I, A and B), intermediate (II), and late (III)[8] (Table 4-1).

Physical Examination

The physical examination may yield normal findings or reveal[9] (1) late systolic bulging at the apex (10% at stage I and about 50% at stages II and III) in left lateral decubitus as an expression of dyskinesis or apical aneurysm with no clinical coronary heart disease; and (2) a palpable presystolic wave (60%), a left S_4 (50%), and, frequently, a giant "a" wave in the jugular venous pulse, data that can be related to early abnormalities in distensibility.

Electrocardiography

The serial ECG study shows the transition from normal to abnormal findings with the appearance of progressive intraventricular conduction disorders. One dominant feature is the frequency and precocity of ventricular arrhythmias, often multifocal and bigeminal. A frequent and very characteristic, although not specific, association is that due to right bundle branch block, left anterior hemiblock, and extrasystolic ventricular arrhythmia (in nearly 50% of patients) (Table 4-2). The stress test shows increased ectopic activity in nearly 30% of patients. Maximum oxygen consumption with exertion is normal during the initial stages. Dynamic, or Holter, ECG allows for a precise study of ventricular arrhythmias and often discloses severe, potentially malignant forms on the basis of the Lown classification. Sustained and nonsustained ventricular tachycardia, idioventricular tachycardia, and ventricular parasystolic rhythm are among the most frequent arrhythmias (Fig. 4-5 and 4-6).

Signal-averaged ECG[11] has shown a high frequency (34% to 42%) of late ventricular potentials in Chagas' cardiomyopathy, closely correlated with arrhythmias in asymptomatic patients with no objective signs of heart disease. These have been attributed to a combination of

Table 4-1.
Clinical Classification of Chagas' Heart Disease

	Symptoms	ECG	Heart size	LVEF	LV wall motion	Autonomic function	Pathologic type
Stage I							
A	None	Normal	Normal	Normal	Normal	Normal	
B	None	Normal	Normal	Normal	Mild abnormalities or diastolic dysfunction	May be abnormal	P-I Concentric
Stage II	Minimal	Conduction abnormalities or VPCs	Normal	Normal	Segmental akinesis or aneurysm	May be abnormal	P-I Concentric
Stage III	CHF, arrhythmias	Conduction abnormalities, pathologic Q waves, complex arrhythmias	Enlarged	Reduced	Global dysfunction with segmental WMA	Usually abnormal	P-II Eccentric

CHF, congestive heart failure; ECG, electrocardiogram; LV, left ventricle; LVEF, left ventricular ejection fraction; P, pathologic type; VPCs, ventricular premature complexes; WMA, wall motion abnormalities.

From Puigbó et al.[8] by permission.

Table 4-2.
Electrocardiographic Findings in Endemic Areas Before and After a Prophylactic Control Program

| | No. of persons studied | Conduction disturbances, % | | | Arrhythmias, VPC, % | Abnormal Q waves, % | PRD, % |
		RBBB	LAFB	LBBB			
Before[8]	1,210	45	26	7	35	10	66
After[10]	1,698	16.8	16.5	⋯	18	⋯	⋯

LAFB, left anterior fascicular block; LBBB, left bundle branch block; PRD, primary repolarization disturbances; RBBB, right bundle branch block; VPC, ventricular premature contraction.

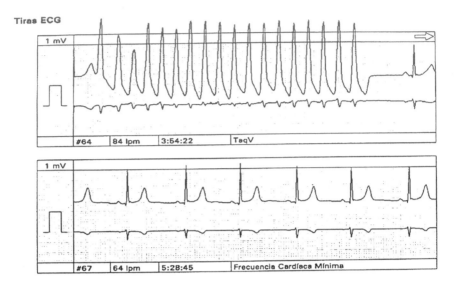

Fig. 4-5. Holter electrocardiographic tracings of sustained ventricular tachycardia in a 40-year-old woman with chronic Chagas' disease. On apical palpation, a late systolic bulging was noticed.

ischemia (due to microcirculation abnormalities with focal areas of hypoperfusion), myocardial fibrosis, and ventricular aneurysms.

Electrophysiologic Studies

Findings on electrophysiologic studies are frequent prolongation of the HV interval and an increase in the His-Purkinje refractory period. The ajmaline test is used to disclose concealed intraventricular conduction disorders.

Echocardiography

Early in the indeterminate phase, the wall motion pattern is normal, and then segmental wall motion abnormalities begin to appear.[10] At stages II or III, about 15% to 20% of patients may have a pattern of hypokinesis of the posterior wall, with preservation of septal motion. This abnormality is related to damage and loss of myocardial fibers and residual fibrosis. Hypertrophic areas, dyskinesis, and, especially, apical aneurysm are frequent findings. The segmental wall motion abnormalities progress to the point of diffuse hypokinesis. Apical dyskinesis progresses until it becomes an apical aneurysm in 50% of patients (Fig. 4-7); it evolves from circumscribed to widespread, with frequent intracavity thrombosis.

Tiras ECG

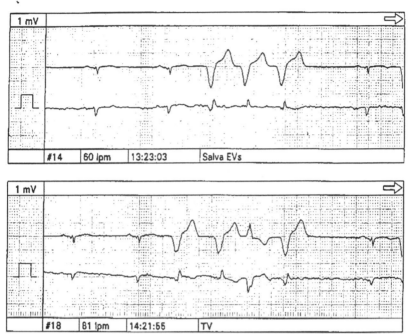

Fig. 4-6. Electrocardiographic recording of nonsustained ventricular tachycardia and multifocal premature ventricular contractions in a 52-year-old man with chronic Chagas' disease. Ventriculography revealed a large apical aneurysm. Electrocardiography also detected a Q-wave pattern (V_1-V_4) (not shown). Eight years earlier, the patient had an embolic cerebrovascular accident.

Echocardiography may disclose intracavity thrombosis (apex and atrial appendages) as a source of systemic and pulmonary emboli, helping to indicate anticoagulation.

Studies[12] have found early alterations of diastolic function, or abnormal relaxation without any impairment of systolic function, as shown by a reduced E:A ratio. In advanced cases, restrictive filling with increased E:A ratio is usually found. Color Doppler scanning allows evaluation of the degree of accompanying mitral and tricuspid regurgitation.

Autonomic dysfunction[13] is often the first and only manifestation of the disease (54%). It becomes evident with abnormalities of the cardiovascular reflexes and with alterations of the heart rate and blood pressure. Autonomic dysfunction is confirmed by pharmacologic and biochemical tests and by studies of heart rate variability (Fig. 4-8 and 4-9).

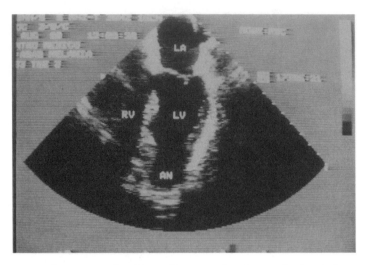

Fig. 4-7. Two-dimensional echocardiogram showing typical apical aneurysm (AN). LA, left atrium; LV, left ventricle; RV, right ventricle.

Radionuclide Angiography and Scintigraphy

Radionuclide angiography makes it possible to evaluate ventricular function and has shown that inferoapical hypokinesis is the most frequently found motion abnormality. This technique also allows visualization of the apical aneurysm.[14] Scintigraphy with thallium 20 has been useful in studying myocardial perfusion.[15] The study at rest and after exercise provides evidence of fixed defects from permanent ischemia or areas of myocardial fibrosis and reversible defects related to transitory ischemia. The perfusion defects are probably related to structural or functional abnormalities of the coronary microvasculature. Scintigraphy with technetium Tc 99m pyrophosphate showed increased uptake in a subgroup of patients studied.[16]

Cardiac Catheterization

Ventriculography studies have made it possible to determine the early onset and progression of segmental wall motion abnormalities, especially in the area of the apex, increased ventricular diastolic volume, decreased distensibility, apical aneurysm, and posterior basal lesion or aneurysm. From intermediate stage II to advanced stage III, ventricular function progressively deteriorates and segmental hypokinesis becomes diffuse hypokinesis. Coronary angiograms show essentially normal epicardial vessels. Nevertheless, an abnormal endothelial coronary response to intracoronary acetylcholine has been found.[17]

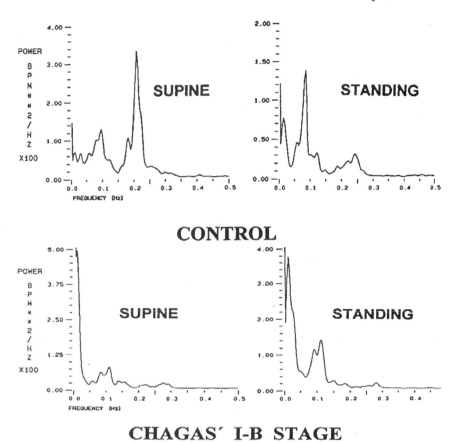

Fig. 4-8. Spectral analysis of the heart rate variability signal in a control subject (panel A) and a patient with stage IB Chagas' disease (panel B). In the patient, the high-frequency component is decreased in both the supine and the standing positions.

Endomyocardial Biopsy

Endomyocardial biopsy has been useful at all phases of the disease. During the acute phase, little fibrosis accompanies the inflammatory process; myocarditis and focal fibrosis are found during the intermediate phase. During the chronic phase, early and progressive myocardial damage is found.[18] Evidence of myocardial lesions is found in 60% of patients with no other evidence of heart disease, in 90% with early contractility abnormalities, in 95% with abnormal ECG findings without heart failure, and in 100% with abnormal ECG findings and heart failure. Polysaccharide deposits with infiltration of the tubular system are found, and there are also reports of immunoglobulin deposits.

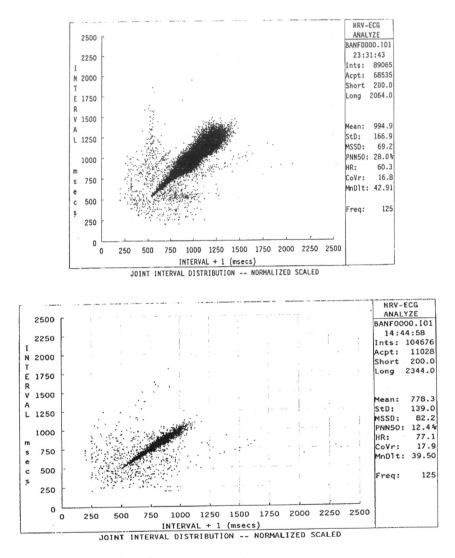

Fig. 4-9. Lorenz plots during a 3-year observation period in a patient with chronic Chagas' disease. Between the first (PNN 50, 28%) and the second (PNN 50, 12.4%) observations, there is deterioration (HRV) accompanied by changes in shape of the plot.

Late Stage III

Clinically, heart failure begins to develop and becomes refractory or progresses to malignant arrhythmias with possible sudden death, the two usual causes of fatal outcome. Less frequently, thromboembolic phenomena occur. In the final stage of the disease, the differential diagnosis becomes dilated (congestive) idiopathic cardiomyopathy. Radiographs show progressive enlargement of the heart. ECGs reveal complex ventricular arrhythmias and atrial fibrillation accompanied by reduced cardiac output. The ECG shows large areas of pathologic Q waves. Complete atrioventricular block and Stokes-Adams attacks are more frequent at this stage. Echocardiograms and cardiac catheterization show an increase in the size of apical aneurysms; there is frequently intracavity thrombosis, with episodes of systemic and pulmonary embolism.

Sudden Death

Chagas' disease is a frequent cause of sudden death, even in young people. In documented cases, sudden death has been due, in most instances, to ventricular fibrillation or, less frequently, to severe bradyarrhythmia. The arrhythmogenic substrata may be related to lesions within the specific conduction tissue. Left ventricular hypertrophy, myocardial inflammation and fibrosis, autonomic dysfunction, microvascular involvement, endothelial dysfunction, ventricular repolarization disorders, and ventricular dysfunction are among the major factors.

Chagas' Disease and AIDS

An association has been found between acquired immunodeficiency syndrome (AIDS) and Chagas' disease. This leads to serious acute infections or to reactivation of chronic infections. Severe neurologic involvement (meningoencephalitis or pseudotumor of the brain) is frequently found. In some patients, *T. cruzi* is acquired through blood transfusions; treatment is an antiparasitic regimen with benznidazole and nifurtimox.

Differential Diagnosis

Two nosologic entities may cause diagnostic problems: dilated (congestive) cardiomyopathy and coronary heart disease (Table 4-3).

Prognosis and Risk Factors

The factors for predicting mortality that had significant statistical value in our series[19] are as follows:

1. *Age*. 56 years or older.
2. *Clinical group*. Asymptomatic or symptomatic (NYHA) grouping has proven to be the most significant predictor of death.

Table 4-3.

Differential Diagnosis: Chronic Chagasic Cardiomyopathy, Dilated Cardiomyopathy, and Coronary Artery Disease

	CV risk factors	Epidemiology	Serology	WMA		Aneurysm		ECG	Autonomic dysfunction	EMB	Coronary angiography	
				S	D	A	O				Ob	ED
CCC	– or +	+	+	+	+	+	+	RBBB LAFB VPC	Early	+	–	+
DC	– or +	–	–	–	+	–	–	LBBB	Late	– or ±	–	+
CAD	+	–	–	+	+	+	+	Var	Late	–	+	+

A, apical; CAD, coronary artery disease; CCC, chronic chagasic cardiomyopathy; CV, cardiovascular; D, diffuse; DC, dilated cardiomyopathy; ECG, electrocardiogram; ED, endothelial dysfunction; EMB, endomyocardial biopsy; LAFB, left anterior fascicular block; LBBB, left bundle branch block; O, other; Ob, obstructive; RBBB, right bundle branch block; S, segmental; Var, variable; VPC, ventricular premature contraction; WMA, wall motion abnormalities.

Patients with ICC have few chances (38% ± 8%) of surviving over an observation period of up to 5 years.

3. *Heart size.* Cardiothoracic ratio 0.50 or greater.
4. *ECG.* Statistically significant predictive variables are chronic atrial fibrillation, extrasystolic ventricular arrhythmia (six or more ventricular premature contractions), and conduction disorders: atrioventricular block (first and second degree and complete), primary repolarization disturbances with left anterior fascicular block, precordial ST-segment elevation, and left ventricular hypertrophy.
5. *Echocardiography.* Ejection fraction, mitral E-septum separation (> 22 mm), left ventricular mass, r:t (radius to thickness) ratio in M mode, internal dimensions of the VI (end-diastolic and end-systolic).
6. *Cineventriculography.* Patients with abnormal ECGs and without ICC have a 10-year survival rate of 65%; the survival rate is only 9% for those with congestive heart failure.[20] In another study performed in the United States, with a follow-up of 53 ± 63 months, the survival rate after 4 years was 56% ± 12%.[1] Survival rates were poor in patients with ventricular dysfunction (left or global) or apical aneurysm.

Control and Treatment

Chagas' disease is linked to underdevelopment and poor social and economic conditions that prevail in a great many rural areas on the American continent. Among the general measures aimed at overcoming these conditions, two specific measures have proven effective: programs aimed at changing the types of dwellings in rural areas and programs aimed at eradicating the vector with insecticides to control transmission of the disease.

The guidelines for treating Chagas' heart disease are

1. Specific antiparasitic drugs, essentially useful in the acute phase, as mentioned above (benznidazole, nifurtimox).
2. Pharmacologic therapy for arrhythmias (amiodarone is especially useful) and implantable cardioverter-defibrillators and pacemakers for long-term treatment of bradyarrhythmias (see the respective chapters).
3. Aneurysmectomies, in selected patients, to control malignant ventricular tachycardia.
4. Conventional treatment of heart failure.
5. Anticoagulants to prevent thromboembolic episodes when intracavity thrombosis or atrial fibrillation is present.
6. Cardiac transplantation for end-stage cardiac disease has been successful. Reactivation of Chagas' disease by immunosuppressive therapy requires antiparasitic drugs.

References

1. Hagar JM, Rahimtoola SH: Chagas' heart disease in the United States. N Engl J Med 325:763-768, 1991
2. Storino R, Milei J: Enfermedad de Chagas, 1993
3. Ben Younés-Chennoufi A, Hontebeyrie-Joskowicz M, Tricottet V, Eisen H, Reynes M, Said G: Persistence of *Trypanosoma cruzi* antigens in the inflammatory lesions of chronically infected mice. Trans R Soc Trop Med Hyg 82:77-83, 1988
4. Jones EM, Colley DG, Tostes S, Lopes ER, Vnencak-Jones CL, McCurley TL: Amplification of a *Trypanosoma cruzi* DNA sequence from inflammatory lesions in human chagasic cardiomyopathy. Am J Trop Med Hyg 48:348-357, 1993
5. Suárez C, Puigbó JJ, Giordano H, Acquatella H, Combellas I, Gómez JR: Ultimos avances de la patología cardíaca chagásica. Rev Fac Med (Caracas) 17:35-56, 1994
6. Parada H, Carrasco HA, Anez N, Fuenmayor C, Inglessis I: Cardiac involvement is a constant finding in acute Chagas' disease: a clinical, parasitological and histopathological study. Int J Cardiol 60:49-54, 1997
7. Lopes ER, Chapadeiro E, Rocha A: Anatomia patológica do coração na forma indeterminada. *In* Cardiopatia Chagásica. Edited by J Romeu Cançado, M Chuster. Belo Horizonte, Fundação Carlos Chagas, 1985
8. Puigbó JJ, Giordano H, Suárez C, Acquatella H, Combellas I: Aspectos clínicos en la enfermedad de Chagas. *In* Actualizaciones en la Enfermedád de Chagas. Edited by RJ Madoery, C Madoery, MI Cámera. Buenos Aires, Organismo Oficial del Congreso Nacional de Medicina, 1993, pp 27-38
9. Giordano H, Puigbó JJ, Acquatella H, Combellas I, Valecillos R, Casal H, Arreaza N, Hirschhaut E, Mendoza I, Tortoledo F, Ferrer I: Miocarditis chagásica: diagnóstico precoz. *In* Miocardiopatías. Edited by H Acquatella, PA Pulido. Barcelona, E Salvat, 1982, pp 43-49
10. Acquatella H, Schiller NB, Puigbó JJ, Giordano H, Suarez JA, Casal H, Arreaza N, Valecillos R, Hirschhaut E: M-mode and two-dimensional echocardiography in chronic Chagas' heart disease. A clinical and pathologic study. Circulation 62:787-799, 1980
11. Madoery C, Guindo J, Esparza E, Viñolas X, Zareba W, Martínez A, Mautner B, Madoery R, Breithardt G, Bayes de Luna A: Signal-averaged ECG in Chagas disease: incidence of late potentials and relationship to cardiac involvement (abstract). J Am Coll Cardiol 19 Suppl:324A, 1992
12. Combellas I, Puigbó JJ, Acquatella H, Tortoledo F, Gomez JR: Echocardiographic features of impaired left ventricular diastolic function in Chagas's heart disease. Br Heart J 53:298-309, 1985
13. Puigbó JJ, Giordano H, Iosa D: Chagas' cardioneuropathy: cardiovascular autonomic dysfunction as the first manifestation of the disease. Int J Angiol 7:123-129, 1998
14. Arreaza N, Puigbó JJ, Acquatella H, Casal H, Giordano H, Valecillos R, Mendoza I, Perez JF, Hirschhaut E, Combellas I: Radionuclide evaluation of left-ventricular function in chronic Chagas' cardiomyopathy. J Nucl Med 24:563-567, 1983
15. Hagar JM, Tubau JF, Rahimtoola SH: Chagas heart disease in the USA: thallium abnormalities mimic coronary artery disease (abstract). Circulation 84 Suppl 2:II-631, 1991

16. da Rocha AF, Meguerian BA, Harbert JC: Tc-99m pyrophosphate myocardial scanning in Chagas' disease. J Nucl Med 22:347-348, 1981

17. Torres FW, Acquatella H, Condado J, Dinsmore R, Palacios IF: Endothelium dependent coronary vasomotion is abnormal in patients with Chagas heart disease (abstract). J Am Coll Cardiol 21 Suppl:197A, 1993

18. Carrasco Guerra HA, Palacios-Pru E, Dagert de Scorza C, Molina C, Inglessis G, Mendoza RV: Clinical, histochemical, and ultrastructural correlation in septal endomyocardial biopsies from chronic chagasic patients: detection of early myocardial damage. Am Heart J 113:716-724, 1987

19. Rodriguez-Salas LA, Klein E, Acquatella H, Catalioti F, Davalos V, Gomez-Mancebo JR, Gonzalez H, Bosch F, Puigbó JJ: Echocardiographic and clinical predictors of mortality in chronic Chagas' disease. Echocardiography 15:271-277, 1998

20. Espinosa R, Carrasco HA, Belandria F, Fuenmayor AM, Molina C, Gonzalez R, Martinez O: Life expectancy analysis in patients with Chagas' disease: prognosis after one decade (1973-1983). Int J Cardiol 8:45-56, 1985

Chapter 5

Effects of Chagas' Disease on Cardiac Autonomic Reflex Function

Carlos A. Morillo, M.D.

Alterations in autonomic innervation both at the central nervous system level and at the peripheral level, including the cardiovascular system, have long been described in Chagas' disease. In 1911, only 2 years after Chagas' disease was first described, Vianna[1] observed nerve lesions in the acute phase of the disease. This damage affected the entire central nervous system, including the cerebellum, medulla oblongata, and spinal cord. Chagas and Villela, in 1922,[2] documented functional compromise of cardiovascular reflex modulation. These investigators noted impaired heart rate response to atropine in patients affected by American trypanosomiasis. Occasionally, some patients experienced negative chronotropic effects after the administration of atropine. Shortening of a baseline prolonged atrioventricular conduction (PR interval) after the administration of atropine suggested that the alterations in atrioventricular node conduction were predominantly related to vagal modulation. Similarly, these investigators suggested that chest pain, frequently observed in chagasic patients, was possibly related to lesions in the sensory nerves of the heart. These observations have been taken as the cornerstone for development of cardiac reflex modulation research in patients with Chagas' disease.

The role of cardiac autonomic dysfunction in the pathogenesis of Chagas' cardiomyopathy remains a matter of debate. Indeed, the pathogenesis of chagasic cardiomyopathy is multifactorial, and cardioneuropathy seems to be important in the development of both conduction and rhythm disturbances frequently observed during the course of the disease. This chapter briefly reviews the pathophysiology and

From Tentori MC, Segura EL, Hayes DL (eds.) *Arrhythmia Management in Chagas' Disease.* Armonk, NY: Futura Publishing Co., Inc. ©2000.

assessment of cardiac autonomic function in patients with different stages of Chagas' cardiomyopathy.

Anatomical Alterations

Several anatomical studies have been published since the description of Chagas' disease. In 1924, Mönberg[3] described the destruction of cardiac ganglionic nerves and cells in a canine model of acute Chagas' disease. Acute Chagas' cardiomyopathy has been associated with both neuronal and ganglionic damage, and inflammatory cellular infiltration has been documented in the perineurium of epicardial cells.[4] Some investigators have suggested that these alterations may be related to the chest pain frequently reported by chagasic patients. Severe compromise of ganglia in the fatty pads has also been associated with rhythm disturbances. In 1958, Köberle[5] described marked degeneration and disappearance of ganglionic cells in acute Chagas' cardiomyopathy. In summary, severe ganglionic degeneration in the subepicardial ganglia of the right atrium with marked reduction in the number of neurons during the acute cardiomyopathy phase has been described. It remains unclear, however, whether these lesions are related simply to the acute inflammatory process, such as subpericarditis, periganglionitis, and ganglionitis, rather than to the direct action of the parasite (*Trypanosoma cruzi*).

Similar findings during the chronic stage of Chagas' cardiomyopathy have also been reported by several investigators. Köberle[6] and Alcántara[7] proposed the "neurotoxin" hypothesis in 1959. These investigators suggested that Chagas' disease is a cardioneuropathy that results from denervation caused by widespread destruction of parasympathetic neurons and nerve fibers at different levels. This hypothesis was based on two primary principles: that parasympathetic nerve destruction is associated with a relative increase in sympathetic activity and that a neurotoxic substance leads to neuronal damage.

Support for the hypothesis was derived from anatomicopathologic studies that evidenced the existence of extensive areas of intrinsic denervation in various organs with typical alterations related to Chagas' disease.[8] Marked reduction of ganglionic cells in the intrinsic nervous system of all organs studied, including the heart, showed definite signs of parasympathetic denervation or neuron loss.[9-11] These findings appear to be distinctive of Chagas' cardiomyopathy. Amorim and Olsen[12] reported greater reduction in cardiac ganglia in Chagas' cardiomyopathy than in dilated cardiomyopathy, providing further support to the "neurogenic" hypothesis (Fig. 5-1).

Chagas' cardioneuropathy has been characterized by marked parasympathetic denervation associated with increased sympathetic drive. However, in 1970, Alcántara[13] reported denervation of intramural ganglia of the heart and cervicothoracic ganglia secondary to Chagas' disease. This finding indicated that both the parasympathetic and the

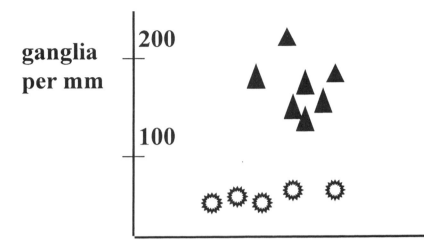

Fig. 5-1. Concentration of cardiac ganglia per millimeter from seven hearts with idiopathic cardiomyopathy (*triangles*) and five hearts with chronic Chagas' cardiomyopathy (*circles*). A marked decrease in the concentration of cardiac ganglia is noted in chagasic hearts. (Adapted from Amorim et al.[12] By permission of the BMJ Publishing Group.)

cervical sympathetic branches could be affected by Chagas' disease, a refutation of the sympathetic hyperactivity hypothesis. Hence, the evaluation of cardiac reflex function becomes of paramount importance to determine the level of alteration of cardiac autonomic modulation. As previously noted, Chagas and Villela[2] observed in 1922 that atropine hardly increased heart rate in patients with chronic Chagas' cardiomyopathy.

Amorim et al.[14] in 1968 and Neto et al.[15] in 1975 pioneered the functional study of cardiac autonomic reflexes in Chagas' cardiomyopathy. These researchers assessed the responses of heart rate and blood pressure either to infusions of vasopressor agents[14] or to postural changes.[15] Both groups arrived at similar conclusions, indicating combined derangement of sympathetic and vagal cardiac reflex responses that vary depending on the degree of cardiomyopathy. These findings also indicate that impaired cardiac reflex function in Chagas' cardiomyopathy is present in the early asymptomatic stages of the disease and is not related to the progression of heart failure.

Pathophysiology

Neural and ganglionic destruction begins during the acute phase and appears to consolidate during the chronic stages of the disease. Neurolysis starts during the acute phase and is provoked by rupture of the "pseudocyst," with consequent liberation of the parasites.[16] This process may destroy up to 80% of the neural structures of the heart and a large proportion of the Auerbach plexus.

It is still unknown whether the direct cytolytic action of substances secreted by the parasite or abnormal immune activation determines neural destruction. A neuraminidase produced by the trypomastigote of *T. cruzi* capable of provoking cellular glycoprotein membrane destruction of myocytes and endothelial cells, leading to cellular destruction, has also been reported.[17] Cellular damage mediated by the immune system is thought to be responsible for alterations observed during the chronic phase of the disease. It has been shown that T lymphocytes from patients with chronic chagasic disease produce and secrete glycoprotein and prostaglandin E_2. Similarly, serum obtained from patients with chronic Chagas' cardiomyopathy carries antilaminin antibodies that by an uncertain mechanism may modulate cholinergic cardiac receptors[18] as well as interact with both muscarinic and β-adrenergic cardiac receptors.[8] These findings suggest that a direct neurolytic effect associated with an abnormal immune response triggered by both acute and chronic inflammation may be related to cardiac neuropathy in Chagas' cardiomyopathy.

Cardiac Reflex Function in Chagas' Cardiomyopathy

Chagas' disease appears to be a unique model of cardioneuropathy. This assumption is based primarily on the characteristics of cardiac reflex function evaluated by noninvasive methods in the different stages of chagasic cardiomyopathy. According to recommendations by the World Health Organization, Chagas' cardiomyopathy may be classified as follows: Chagas' 1, asymptomatic with normal findings on electrocardiography (ECG) and chest radiography; Chagas' 2, asymptomatic with normal chest x-ray findings and mild ECG abnormalities, such as right bundle branch block, hemiblocks, sinus bradycardia, and premature ventricular complexes; and Chagas' 3, dilated cardiomyopathy with heart failure and ECG abnormalities that include atrioventricular block and nonsustained and sustained ventricular tachycardia.

Several studies have addressed the issue of altered cardiac reflex function in different stages of the disease. The importance of preserved cardiac reflex function has recently been emphasized by several studies that indicated that impaired cardiovagal reflexes are associated with a higher risk of sudden cardiac death and overall cardiac mortality after acute myocardial infarction.[18]

Heart Rate Response

Sinus bradycardia has been considered one of the clinical features of Chagas' cardiomyopathy. Palmero et al.[19] compared baseline heart rate in 222 chagasic patients with that in 50 healthy controls and 55 subjects with congestive heart failure of other cause. Patients with Chagas' disease without signs of congestive heart failure had lower heart rates than controls, although this difference did not reach statistical significance. On the other hand, chagasic patients with heart failure had a significantly lower heart rate than a matched group of patients with congestive heart failure not related to Chagas' disease. These findings indicate an impaired sinus node response in subjects with Chagas' disease, possibly related to abnormalities in the innervation of the sinus node or, alternatively, to impaired sinus node automaticity.

We recently studied several patients with various degrees of Chagas' cardiomyopathy after pharmacologic testing, including isoproterenol dose response curves and complete sinus node denervation with atropine and propranolol.[20] Our findings indicated that a combination of reduced chronotropic response after isoproterenol bolus infusions and markedly reduced intrinsic heart rate, indicating impaired sinus node automaticity, may be responsible for the bradycardia.

Response to Orthostatic Stress

The maintenance of blood pressure during postural changes is largely regulated by adaptation of sympathetic and vagal baroreflex mechanisms. Response to orthostatic stress by either active standing or passive upright tilting has been promoted as a useful noninvasive method for the evaluation of the integrity of the mentioned reflex mechanisms. Orthostatic intolerance manifested by postural hypotension has long been recognized in patients with Chagas' cardiomyopathy. Palmero et al.[21] studied 115 chagasic patients and documented a lower mean arterial pressure in patients than in controls. Orthostatic intolerance may be associated with syncope in some patients and is characterized by hypotension without reflex tachycardia. This finding is generally attributed to arterial baroreflex dysfunction or impaired catecholamine secretion. Compared with controls and patients with heart failure not related to Chagas' disease, chagasic patients have a lower increase in diastolic pressure and a blunted heart rate response. The mechanism of this response is primarily related to impaired arterial baroreceptor response to orthostatic stress, particularly an impaired baroreflex-mediated sympathetic response that leads to lack of peripheral vasoconstriction with subsequent hypotension. Interestingly, as documented by Palmero et al.,[22] the impaired baroreflex response to orthostatic stress is documented early in the development of the disease during the asymptomatic phase. These findings corroborate the notion that the dysautonomic response observed in Chagas' cardiomyopathy is related to an early involvement of cardiac innervation rather than progression of heart failure.[23,24]

Other noninvasive tests of autonomic function that may evaluate sympathetic or parasympathetic pathways, such as the Valsalva maneuver, deep breathing test, cold pressor test, and cold face test, have been performed during the different stages of Chagas' cardiomyopathy. Our laboratory recently used a battery of autonomic function tests to evaluate 34 seropositive subjects with asymptomatic Chagas' disease, 12 survivors of sudden cardiac arrest with Chagas' cardiomyopathy, and 22 healthy volunteers.[23-25] Subjects were classified according to clinical stage as Chagas' 1 (asymptomatic with normal ECG), Chagas' 2 (asymptomatic with minor ECG abnormalities), or Chagas' 3 (heart failure and sudden cardiac arrest). These findings are discussed in the sections that follow.

Valsalva Maneuver

Analysis of the beat-to-beat changes in heart rate and blood pressure during the compression (phase 2) and overshooting (phase 4) phases of the Valsalva maneuver provides information on the sympathetic and parasympathetic integrity of cardiovascular reflex function. Changes in systolic blood pressure and reflex changes in heart rate during phase 2 of the Valsalva maneuver are proposed as indexes of sympathetic activity. In contrast, phase 4 causes an abrupt increase in systolic blood pressure with a reflex bradycardia that provides information on the response of the arterial baroreflex related to cardiovagal efferent traffic.

Most studies have demonstrated an alteration in both sympathetic and parasympathetic control in patients with Chagas' cardiomyopathy. Asymptomatic carriers have a combined disorder that is progressive and related to Chagas' stage.

Cold Pressor Test

The cold pressor test is a simple method for the functional evaluation of the sympathetic efferent pathway. Immersion of the hand in cold ice water triggers an increase in both systolic and diastolic blood pressure. Reduction of or a blunted response in the increase in blood pressure is observed in subjects with impaired sympathetic efferent response. Similarly, an exaggerated response strongly suggests that the response is mediated by hypersensitivity denervation. The percent change in mean arterial pressure during this maneuver is shown in the three groups of patients with Chagas' disease and in a control group (Fig. 5-2). The response is progressively reduced in patients but not in control subjects, an indication of impaired sympathetic efferent traffic. This finding suggests that reduced β-adrenoreceptor availability or response is progressively impaired by Chagas' cardiomyopathy. Iosa et al.[25] described similar findings but documented a marked increase

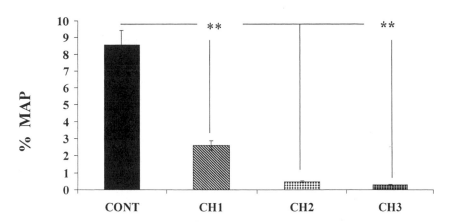

Fig. 5-2. Percent change in mean arterial pressure (MAP) during the cold pressor test. Progressive reduction in systolic pressure change indicates progressive sympathetic involvement. CONT, controls; CH1, Chagas' stage 1; CH2, Chagas' stage 2; CH3, Chagas' stage 3. ¨Clinically significant.

in blood pressure in patients with Chagas' 3 classification, attributing this result to hypersensitivity denervation. An explanation for these differences may be that all our patients in the Chagas' 3 group were also survivors of sudden cardiac arrest, a factor possibly influencing the response to sympathetic efferent stimuli.

The deep breathing and cold face tests, which evaluate both central and peripheral integrity of vagal control, also documented a significant reduction in heart rate response (bradycardia) with vagal stimuli. This impaired response was also progressive and was related to the stage of Chagas' cardiomyopathy.

In summary, all autonomic tests of vagal efferent function showed progressive impairment in the asymptomatic stage. A marked reduction in vagal modulation was noted in survivors of sudden cardiac arrest.[23-26] These markers explore the integrity of tonic modulation of vagal control and indicate that even during the asymptomatic stages, important cardiovagal reflex function is impaired.

Arterial Baroreceptor Sensitivity

Regulation of arterial baroreflex modulation is directly linked to vagal efferent activity and to control of vascular sympathetic activity. The linear correlation between changes in systolic blood pressure and RR interval determines the baroreflex gain or sensitivity. Abrupt changes in blood pressure provoked by infusion of vasoactive agents, such as phenylephrine and nitroprusside, have been widely used to evaluate arterial baroreceptor response. Impaired arterial baroreflex response has recently been identified as a risk marker for global cardiovascular mortality and the appearance of fatal arrhythmic events. This simple maneuver evaluates the phasic modulation of vagal efferent activity.

We recently studied the arterial baroreflex response in 32 asymptomatic carriers and 12 survivors of sudden cardiac arrest with advanced Chagas' cardiomyopathy. A tendency to reduced baroreflex sensitivity was documented in patients with Chagas' 1 and Chagas' 2 classifications. However, this difference did not reach statistical significance. In contrast, markedly reduced baroreflex sensitivity (<2 msec/mm Hg), was documented in all the patients with sudden cardiac arrest (Fig. 5-3). Additionally, ventricular tachycardia associated with hemodynamic collapse or ventricular fibrillation (or both) was induced at electrophysiologic study in all patients. Chagasic patients with an episode of sudden cardiac arrest due to either ventricular tachycardia or ventricular fibrillation have severe impairment of phasic vagal efferent modulation.[25] Iosa[25] also reported significant reductions in baroreflex gain that were progressive with the stage of the disease. To the best of our knowledge, however, Iosa et al. did not explore patients who survived an episode of ventricular tachycardia or fibrillation. Baroreflex sensitivity is severely impaired in patients with Chagas' cardiomyopathy, indicating a markedly reduced phasic response of efferent vagal traffic that may be related to the genesis and modulation of lethal arrhythmias in this situation.

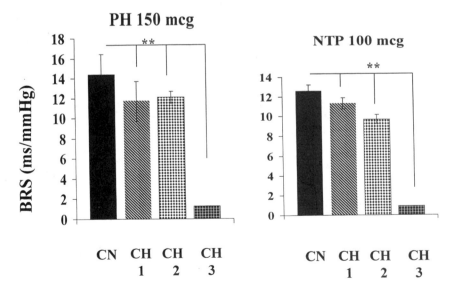

Fig. 5-3. Baroreflex slopes (BRS) to either phenylephrine (PH) or nitroprusside (NTP) bolus injections in patients with different stages (CH1, CH2, CH3) of Chagas' cardiomyopathy. Marked reduction in baroreflex gain is noted in survivors of sudden cardiac arrest (CH3). CN, controls; **P < 0.001.

Heart Rate Variability

Spontaneous changes in beat-to-beat regulation of heart rate are well documented to be related to efferent vagal modulation of the sinus node. These oscillations in heart period (RR interval) may be evaluated in the time or frequency domain and primarily reflect sympathovagal regulation of heart rate. Several studies in patients after myocardial infarction or in patients with heart failure have conclusively validated the importance of these markers as indicators of high risk for cardiac and arrhythmic mortality.[18] Few studies have systematically evaluated heart rate variability in patients with Chagas' cardiomyopathy. Guzzetti et al.[27] published the first report on power spectral analysis of heart rate variability in patients with different stages of chagasic cardiomyopathy. These authors documented impaired activation of low-frequency oscillations (usually accepted as a marker of sympathetic activity modulated by baroreceptor integrity) both at rest and after orthostatic stress, an indication of severe alteration in sympathetic activation and markedly reduced tonic vagal activity. More importantly, the authors established that cardioneuropathy was present even before the development of any cardiovascular symptoms.

In a similar study, we corroborated these findings and additionally proposed that sympathoexcitation is present during the early asymptomatic stage (Chagas' 1) of the disease.[23,24] A marked and progressive reduction in total power spectra (Fig. 5-4) supports the notion that progressive, severe vagal cardioneuropathy appears well before the development of any cardiovascular abnormality. Similarly, we documented initial sympathoexcitation, as evidenced by a shift toward an increased index of low frequency to high frequency (LF/HF) in patients with Chagas' 1 classification followed by a reduced LF/HF index (Fig. 5-5). These findings support the interpretation of early sympathoexcitation followed by progressive loss of tonic and phasic vagal modulation of heart rate. Additionally, we documented marked reduction in the 0.1-Hz oscillations of systolic blood pressure. These oscillations are primarily modulated by baroreceptor function.

In summary, power spectral analysis of heart rate and blood pressure variabilities has consistently documented a progressive reduction in vagal modulation related to the stage of the disease. Similarly, early sympathoexcitation documented in clinically asymptomatic subjects is progressively reduced as the disease progresses. Alterations in baroreceptor gain have also been demonstrated by impaired activation of baroreflex mechanisms induced during both pharmacologic and orthostatic stress.

Treatment of Chagas' Cardioneuropathy

Therapy for cardioneuropathy is currently limited to management of symptoms of autonomic dysfunction. Symptoms of orthostatic intol-

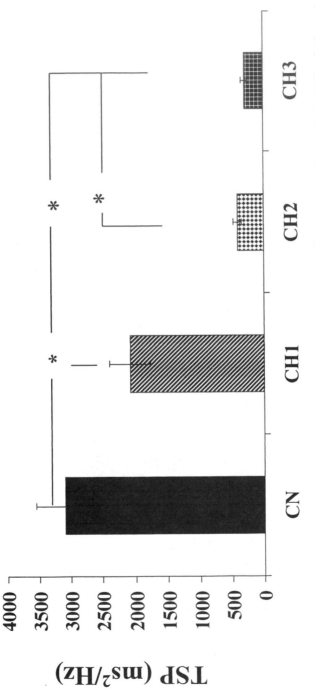

Fig. 5-4. Mean total power spectra (TSP) in controls (CN) and patients with different stages (CH1, CH2, CH3) of Chagas' disease. Significant and progressive reductions in total power indicate alterations in tonic control of heart rate variability. *Clinically significant.

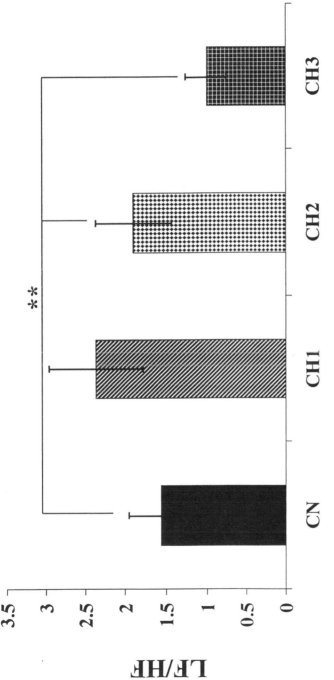

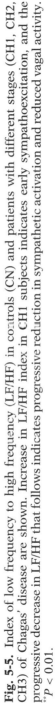

Fig. 5-5. Index of low frequency to high frequency (LF/HF) in controls (CN) and patients with different stages (CH1, CH2, CH3) of Chagas' disease are shown. Increase in LF/HF index in CH1 subjects indicates early sympathoexcitation, and the progressive decrease in LF/HF that follows indicates progressive reduction in sympathetic activation and reduced vagal activity. **P < 0.01.

erance, achalasia, and constipation should be pursued and treated by conventional methods. Specific therapy for chronic chagasic cardioneuropathy was first reported by Iosa.[25] This investigator proposed the use of exogenous ganglioside therapy for the management of chagasic cardioneuropathy. The rationale for the use of gangliosides is based on several findings. First, sufficient evidence supports the importance of cardiac denervation in the pathophysiology of chagasic cardiomyopathy. Second, *T. cruzi* produces a neuraminidase capable of removing sialic acid from glycoproteins, glycolipids, and oligosaccharides. Third, neuraminidase activity shows a 20-fold increase after the trypanosome becomes infective, suggesting that neuraminidase contributes to the pathogenesis of Chagas' disease. Fourth, purified mixtures of gangliosides have been shown to stimulate in vitro and in vivo reinnervation in different neuropathies.

On the basis of these hypothetical mechanisms, Iosa et al.[28] conducted a double-blind, placebo-controlled trial in Argentina and Venezuela to test the hypothesis that Cronassial (a ganglioside) restores cardiac autonomic function in patients with cardioneuropathy and different stages of chagasic cardiomyopathy. In this crossover study, which included 128 patients, Cronassial was compared with a placebo. The main findings were that ganglioside therapy during 4 weeks restored cardiac reflex response, particularly by improving the response to orthostatic stress and the heart rate response to hyperventilation, indications of improved sympathetic and possibly baroreflex functions.

More recently, our group proposed that intravenous β-adrenergic blockade be used to restore cardiac reflexes.[29] On the basis of our findings of early sympathoexcitation with subsequent progressive cardiovagal denervation, we proposed that β-adrenergic blockade (with metoprolol) might restore impaired cardiac reflex activity. To test this hypothesis, we randomly assigned 20 patients to receive metoprolol or placebo intravenously and evaluated a battery of cardiac autonomic function tests before and after the intervention. The main findings were significant increases in most of the time and frequency domain markers of vagal activity after the intravenous administration of metoprolol. Similarly, reduction in both heart period LF oscillations and LF:HF ratio suggested reduced sympathetic activity. Interestingly, a greater compromise of cardiac autonomic function was needed to obtain a greater effect with metoprolol (Fig. 5-6). Further studies are under way to test the efficacy of oral metoprolol during 4 weeks in a crossover, placebo-controlled trial.

In summary, therapy for Chagas' cardioneuropathy remains directed toward symptoms. Recent studies indicate the potential for use of gangliosides (e.g., Cronassial) or β-adrenergic blocking agents in an attempt to restore cardiac reflex function. It remains to be proven whether restoration of cardiac reflexes is associated with improvement in functional status, reduction in arrhythmic events, and delayed progression of chagasic cardiomyopathy.

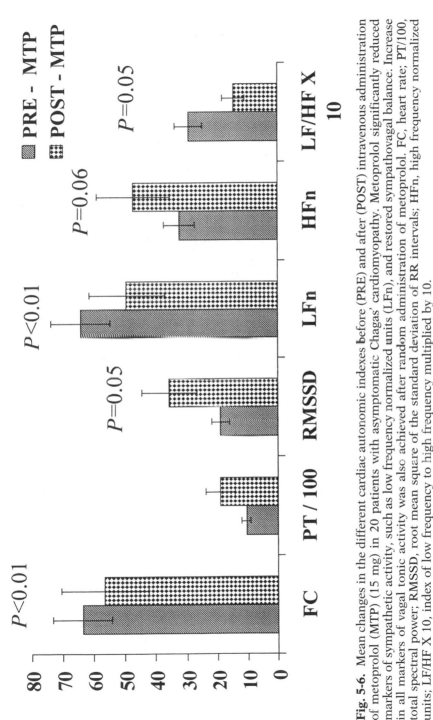

Fig. 5-6. Mean changes in the different cardiac autonomic indexes before (PRE) and after (POST) intravenous administration of metoprolol (MTP) (15 mg) in 20 patients with asymptomatic Chagas' cardiomyopathy. Metoprolol significantly reduced markers of sympathetic activity, such as low frequency normalized units (LFn), and restored sympathovagal balance. Increase in all markers of vagal tonic activity was also achieved after random administration of metoprolol. FC, heart rate; PT/100, total spectral power; RMSSD, root mean square of the standard deviation of RR intervals; HFn, high frequency normalized units; LF/HF X 10, index of low frequency to high frequency multiplied by 10.

Conclusions

Cardiac autonomic dysfunction occurs in 38% to 52% of persons with Chagas' cardiomyopathy, representing a unique model of primary cardioneuropathy. Impairment of cardiac reflex activity is reported early during the asymptomatic stage and becomes severe as the disease stage progresses. To what extent these early alterations contribute to the development of cardiomyopathy is unclear. The role for routine testing of cardiac autonomic function for risk stratification in patients with Chagas' cardiomyopathy remains speculative and requires proof in large longitudinal studies. However, it seems reasonable to presume that information derived from simple cardiac autonomic reflex testing will provide valuable information for the management of patients with Chagas' cardiomyopathy. Eventually, early identification of cardiac autonomic dysfunction may prove to be an early harbinger of Chagas' cardiomyopathy.

Acknowledgment: The author acknowledges the support of an Established Investigator grant from COLCIENCIAS (Colombian Institute for the Advancement of Science and Technology).

References

1. Vianna C: Contribuição para estudo da anatomia patolojica da "molestia de Carlos Chagas." Mem Inst Oswaldo Cruz iii:276-294, 1911
2. Chagas C, Villela E: Forma cardiaca da trypanosomiase americana. Mem Inst Oswaldo Cruz xiv:5-61, 1922
3. Mönberg JG: Die Erkrandunges des myokards und des spezifischen muskelsystems. *In* Handbuch Spezial Pathologisch Anatomie un Histologie. Berlin, Springer, 1924
4. Torres CM, Duarte E: Miocardite na forma aguda da doenca de Chagas. Mem Inst Oswaldo Cruz 46:759-793, 1948
5. Köberle F: Cardiopatia chagásica. Hospital (Rio J) 53:311-346, 1958
6. Köberle F: Aspectos neurológicos da meléstia de Chagas. Arch Neuropsiquitr 25:159-174, 1967
7. Alcántara FG: Sistema neurovegetativo do coracao na moléstia de Chagas experimental. Rev Goiana Med 7:111-126, 1961
8. Lázzari JO: Autonomic nervous system alterations in Chagas disease: review of the literature. *In* Chagas and the Nervous System. Washington, Panamerican Health Organization. 547:72-96, 1994
9. Alencar A: The autonomic nervous system of the heart in experimental infestation of the albino mouse with *Schizotrypanum cruzi* [Portuguese]. Arq Bras Med 50:95-102, 1960
10. Tafuri WL: Lesoes do sistema nervoso autónomo do coracao e do colo do camundongo na fase aguda da doenca de Chagas experimental; estudios ao microscópio ótico e ao electrónico. Rev Asoc Med Minas Gerais 19:3-39, 1968

11. Lopes ER, Tafuri WL, Bogliolo L, Almeida HO, Chapadeiro E, Raso P: Acute human Chagasic myocarditis (sub-epicardial ganglionitis: lymphocytic aggression to the cardiac fibers; relation between amastigota and muscle fibers [Portuguese]. Rev Inst Med Trop Sao Paulo 19:301-309, 1977

12. Amorim DS, Olsen EG: Assessment of heart neurons in dilated (congestive) cardiomyopathy. Br Heart J 47:11-18, 1982

13. Alcántara FG: Alteracoes morfológicas e histoquímicas dos neuronios parasimpáticos cardíacos e dos simpáticos dos ganglios cervicotorácicos na moléstia de Chagas. Rev Goiana Med 17:1-17, 1971

14. Amorim DS, Godoy RA, Manco JC, Tanaka A, Gallo L Jr: Effects of acute elevation in blood pressure and of atropine on heart rate in Chagas' disease. A preliminary report. Circulation 38:289-294, 1968

15. Neto JA, Gallo L Jr, Manco JC, Rassi A, Amorim DS: Postural reflexes in chronic Chagas's heart disease. Heart rate and arterial pressure responses. Cardiology 60:343-357, 1975

16. Ferreira-Berrutti P: Evolución normal y patológica de los nidos parasitarios en las fibras miocárdicas humanas en la enfermedad de Chagas. Arch Soc de Biol de Montevideo 11:101-107, 1943

17. Iosa D, Dequattro V, Lee DD, Elkayam U, Caeiro T, Palmero H: Pathogenesis of cardiac neuro-myopathy in Chagas' disease and the role of the autonomic nervous system. J Auton Nerv Syst 30 Suppl:S83-S87, 1990

18. La Rovere MT, Bigger JT Jr, Marcus FI, Mortara A, Schwartz PJ, for the ATRAMI (Autonomic Tone and Reflexes After Myocardial Infarction) Investigators: Baroreflex sensitivity and heart-rate variability in prediction of total cardiac mortality after myocardial infarction. Lancet 351:478-484, 1998

19. Palmero HA, Caeiro TF, Iosa D: Prevalence of slow heart rates in chronic Chagas' disease. Am J Trop Med Hyg 30:1179-1182, 1981

20. Morillo CA, Villar JC, Nino J: Chagasic cardiomyopathy: a unique model of cardiac autonomic dysfunction. Arch Maladies du Coeur 91:100, 1998

21. Palmero HA, Caeiro TF, Iosa DJ: Effect of Chagas' discase on arterial blood pressure. Am Heart J 97:38-42, 1979

22. Palmero HA, Caeiro TF, Iosa DJ: Distinctive abnormal responses to tilting test in chronic Chagas' disease. Klin Wochenschr 58:1307-1311, 1980

23. Villar JC, Morillo CA Vega A, et al: Cambios en la función autonómica cardíaca en sujetos seropositivos a T. cruzi asintomáticos. Rev Col Cardiol 6:7-14, 1997

24. Villar JC, León H, Contreras JP, Amado PM, Pradilla LP, Tahvanainen KUO, Eckberg DL, Morillo CA: Cardiac autonomic dysfunction in asymptomatic subjects with positive Chagas' serology (abstract). Circulation 94 Suppl:I-313, 1996

25. Iosa D: Chronic chagasic cardioneuropathy: pathogenesis and treatment. In Chagas and the Nervous System. Washington, Panamerican Health Organization. 547:99-148, 1994

26. Villar JC, Niño J, Amado PM, Tahvanainen KUO, Kuusela T, Morillo CA: Impaired cardiac reflexes and increased QT-dispersion in sudden cardiac death survivors with Chagas' cardiomyopathy (abstract). Eur Heart J 19 Suppl:246, 1998

27. Guzzetti S, Iosa D, Pecis M, Bonura L, Prosdocimi M, Malliani A: Impaired heart rate variability in patients with chronic Chagas' disease. Am Heart J 121:1727-1734, 1991

28. Iosa D, Massari DC, Dorsey FC: Chagas' cardioneuropathy: effect of gangli-oside treatment in chronic dysautonomic patients—a randomized, double-blind, parallel, placebo-controlled study. Am Heart J 122:775-785, 1991
29. Villar JC, Amado PM, Niño J, Tahvanainen KUO, Morillo CA: Tonic vagal activity is increased by metoprolol in asymptomatic Chagas' positive serol-ogy subjects (abstract). Clin Auton Res 9:66, 1999

Chapter 6

Signal-Averaged Electrocardiography in Chagas' Disease

Cristián Madoery, M.D.,
Aurora Ruiz, M.D.
Antonio Martínez-Rubio, M.D.,
Roberto Madoery, M.D.,

Worldwide, between 20 and 30 million persons are affected by Chagas' disease, and more than 90 million are at risk of infection by living in endemic areas.[1] In Central and South America, particularly Brazil, Argentina, Venezuela, and Chile, Chagas' disease is one of the main public health concerns.[1] Although it is traditionally thought that Chagas' disease is a rare event in the United States, its prevalence has been shown to be considerably higher than expected.[2]

The main cardiovascular indicator is cardiomyopathy, which is observed some years after the initial infection. From 20% to 25% of infected patients present with cardiac manifestations, including cardiac enlargement, congestive heart failure, intraventricular conduction disturbances, ventricular arrhythmias, and sudden cardiac arrest.[3,4] Syncope and sudden death due to ventricular fibrillation are a continuous threat and may be the first indication of the disease.[5] In Argentina alone, Chagas' disease accounts for 5,000 to 6,000 deaths every year, half of which are sudden, due to tachyarrhythmias or bradyarrhythmias.[6] Despite the high prevalence and incidence of sudden death, very few studies have been carried out to analyze the potential risk predictors of complex ventricular arrhythmias and sudden death in patients with Chagas' disease.

From Tentori MC, Segura EL, Hayes DL (eds.) *Arrhythmia Management in Chagas' Disease.* Armonk, NY: Futura Publishing Co., Inc. ©2000.

Over the past few years, a number of researchers have used the signal-averaging technique to record high-frequency, low-amplitude signals occurring at the end of the QRS complex or in the ST segment.[7,8] These signals, usually called "ventricular late potentials," originate in tissue zones in which viable muscle alternates with necrotic or fibrotic muscular tissue. Late potentials are considered markers of an arrhythmogenic substrate that, under certain conditions (e.g., triggering factors such as ventricular premature complex), may cause sustained ventricular tachyarrhythmias. The recording techniques, pathophysiologic mechanisms, and prognostic value of these signals have been widely reported, particularly in patients with coronary artery disease.[7-10] On the contrary, only a few reports exist on these techniques in patients with Chagas' disease, and information on long-term prognosis is particularly lacking.[11-13]

Some groups have shown the existence of an electrophysiologic substrate for ventricular tachycardia in patients with chagasic cardiomyopathy.[5,14] These events have led us to investigate the potential of signal-averaged electrocardiography (SAECG) in the early diagnosis of myocardial involvement. The purpose of our study, therefore, was to prospectively evaluate the prevalence of abnormal findings on SAECG and their prognostic value as a marker of lethal ventricular tachyarrhythmias in patients with Chagas' disease.

Recording Techniques

Late potentials have an amplitude of a few millivolts if they are registered in situ during catheter-based endocardial mapping or during epicardial or endocardial intraoperative mapping.[15] These potentials can seldom be registered from the body surface by conventional methods. That is why a wide amplification of signals, bidirectional filters, and computerized averaging techniques are needed.

Two techniques are commonly used to register late potentials. The time domain technique is not only the most widely used but also the only one with standardized positivity criteria.[7,8] It is based on amplification; signal filtering and the average of a certain number of similar beats enable the elimination of noise (Fig. 6-1). This method is useful only in patients with narrow QRS (<120 msec).

The other technique is analysis in the frequency domain, which uses the fast Fourier transform, in which the outcome signal is mathematically decomposed and analyzed by its sinusoidal components (harmonic).[16,17] Cain et al.[16] showed that the terminal portion of QRS of high-frequency components was increased in patients with ventricular arrhythmia (88%) in comparison to those without arrhythmia (15%) between the frequencies of 20 and 50 Hz (Fig. 6-2).

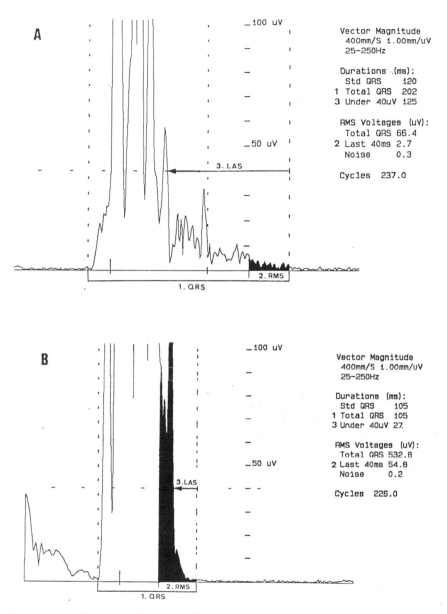

Fig. 6-1. *A,* Electrocardiogram of averaged signal in time domain in a 50-year-old man with Chagas' disease and a clinical history of sustained ventricular tachycardia. *B,* Electrocardiogram of averaged signal in time domain in a 48-year-old woman with Chagas' disease and without signs of complex ventricular arrhythmia.

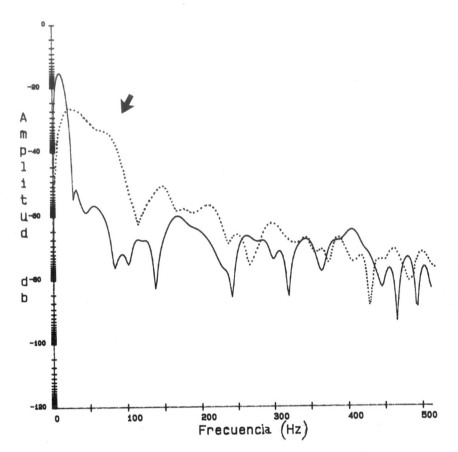

Fig. 6-2. Spectral representation in frequency domain analysis of the terminal portion of the QRS and the ST segment in two chagasic patients who have complete bundle branch block, one with sustained ventricular tachycardia (*dotted line*) and the other without a history of ventricular tachycardia (*continuous line*). An abnormal contribution is shown by high-frequency components (*arrow*).

SAECG After Myocardial Infarction

The SAECG technique has been studied most thoroughly in patients who have had myocardial infarction.[7-10] Simson,[7] in a study with SAECG during the first month after infarction, found a prevalence of ventricular tachycardia between 24% and 44%.

SAECG is considered a very specific method (around 90%) because it does not detect late ventricular activity in patients without it during intraoperative mapping. Its sensitivity is somehow lower (70% to 80%), because late activation cannot be detected from the body surface in patients in whom it can be detected during epicardial mapping. The predictive positive value is low (15% to 20%), but the predictive negative value is very high (95% to 99%).[8-10]

To increase the predictive value of predictors of sustained ventricular tachycardia or sudden death after acute myocardial infarction, several prospective studies have assessed the value of the association of different diagnostic methods, such as SAECG, 24-hour Holter recording, and isotopic ventriculography.[10] All studies agree that although an abnormal SAECG result is an independent factor, maximum predictive value is reached when other diagnostic techniques are also performed. In 1992, Steinberg et al.[9] studied 182 patients after myocardial infarction and found that SAECG results were abnormal in about 39%. The negative predictive value was 95%, and the positive predictive value was 15%. Abnormal SAECG findings in addition to detection of arrhythmias on Holter monitoring increased the risk to 26% (compared with 4% if results of both studies were normal).

SAECG in Patients With Cardiomyopathies

Although most of the studies of SAECG were done in patients after myocardial infarction, several were completed in patients with different cardiomyopathies (e.g., hypertrophic and dilated cardiomyopathies and arrhythmogenic right ventricular dysplasia).[8,18-20]

Poll et al.[18] found that in patients with nonischemic dilated cardiomyopathy who had a history of malignant arrhythmias, the prevalence of abnormal SAECG findings was about 83%, whereas only 14% of patients without documentation of malignant arrhythmias had abnormal SAECG results. Middlekauff et al.[19] determined that the prevalence of abnormal findings on SAECG was higher in patients with dilated cardiomyopathy of ischemic origin (40%) than in patients with cardiomyopathy of nonischemic origin (14%). Nevertheless, abnormal SAECG results in patients with nonischemic cardiomyopathy were not associated with an increase in the risk of sudden death.

In hypertrophic cardiomyopathy, the prevalence of abnormal SAECG findings is from 8% to 20%, and, in general, no positive predictive value for malignant events is found.[20]

SAECG in Chagas' Disease

Although several groups are currently studying late potentials in Chagas' disease, only a few results have been published to date.[11-13,21] In 1990, a multicenter study was started in Argentina to determine the prevalence of abnormal SAECG findings in Chagas' disease, the relationship to different degrees of cardiac involvement, and the predictive value.[12,21]

Characteristics of Patients

Eighty-four consecutive patients (25 male, 59 female) with a serologic finding positive for *Trypanosoma cruzi* were prospectively evaluated by two of the following methods: Machado-Guerreiro test, complement fixation test, and immunofluorescence.[3,22] The mean age of the study population was 49 ± 16 years. Patients with coronary artery disease were excluded. The patients were divided into four groups:

Group A: 24 patients in whom cardiac damage was not detected.

Group B: 29 patients with abnormal findings on the surface electrocardiogram (ECG) or 24-hour Holter recording (or both) but with an ejection fraction greater than 50%.

Group C: 12 patients in New York Heart Association (NYHA) functional class 2 or higher or with an abnormal ventricular ejection fraction (or both) but with normal findings on the surface ECG and Holter recording.

Group D: 19 patients with abnormal findings on the surface ECG or Holter recording (or both) and an NYHA functional class of 2 or higher or an abnormal ejection fraction (or both).

The results of SAECG in patients with Chagas' disease were compared with those in a group of 40 healthy persons with no evidence of cardiac disease on routine examination. The control group did not live in areas endemic for Chagas' disease.

Twenty-four of the 84 patients (29%) were asymptomatic and had no signs of structural myocardiopathy or arrhythmias (group A). Sixty of the 84 patients (71%) satisfied one or more anomalous criteria (groups B, C, and D). Table 6-1 shows the clinical characteristics of the patients in each group. Twenty-four patients (29%) were in NYHA functional class 2 or higher, and 35 patients (42%) had conduction disturbances on the surface ECG. Sixteen patients (19%) had a cardiothoracic index greater than 50% on the chest radiograph. The average left ventricular ejection fraction by echocardiography was 55.6%; 31 patients (37%) had an ejection fraction of less than 50%. Twenty-nine patients (34%) had frequent ventricular premature contractions, and 15 patients (18%) had couplets and runs of ventricular tachycardia on the initial 24-hour Holter recording.

SAECG Methods

The signals of three orthogonal leads were recorded, averaged, and analyzed in time domain and in frequency domain with commercially available equipment.

Time domain analysis was performed with a bidirectional filter of 40 to 250 Hz. The SAECG result was considered to be abnormal if

Table 6-1.
Characteristics of Patients

Group	Age, yr*	F/M, no.	CTI, %*	IVCD, no.	LVDD, mm*	EF, %*	VPC (24 hr), no.*	VPC (>10/hr), no.	Couplets and runs, no.
A	38 ± 3	17/7	43 ± 4	0	44 ± 5	66 ± 11	5 ± 14	0	0
B	54 ± 1	21/8	45 ± 5	21	45 ± 6	65 ± 8	1,407 ± 2,962	15	5
C	45 ± 6	9/3	49 ± 4	0	51 ± 15	37 ± 7	9 ± 31	0	0
D	56 ± 15	12/7	54 ± 6	14	54 ± 10	41 ± 15	4,743 ± 7,445	14	10
	49 ± 16	59/25	48 ± 5	35	48 ± 11	56 ± 12	1,561 ± 3,067	29	15

CTI, cardiothoracic index; EF, left ventricular ejection fraction; F/M, female/male; IVCD, intraventricular conduction disturbances; LVDD, left ventricular diastolic diameters; VPC, ventricular premature contractions.
*Mean ± standard deviation.

two or more of the following criteria were met: (1) total filtered QRS duration > 114 msec, (2) average voltage of the last 40 msec (root-mean-square 40) < 20 μV, and (3) duration of low-amplitude signals (< 40 μV) in the final portion of the QRS (low-amplitude signal) > 38 msec (see Fig. 6-1).

For analysis in frequency domain,[8,16,17] 512-point fast Fourier transform was performed using a 120-msec segment of each of the averaged leads (X, Y, Z). The segment under analysis began 20 msec before the end of the QRS complex and was multiplied point-by-point with use of a special window (Blackmann-Harris) to reduce spectral leakage (Fig. 6-2). Three different area ratios (ARs) were analyzed to evaluate whether high-frequency components were present: AR I = 20-50/0-20 Hz;[16] AR II = 60-120/0-30 Hz; and AR III = 50-150/0-30 Hz.[17] The following ARs were considered abnormal:[17] AR I, ≥275; AR II, ≥80; and AR III, ≥140. The SAECG result was considered to be abnormal when two or more ARs had abnormal values, indicating high-frequency components.

The spectral turbulence analysis technique uses an algorithm defining an area that starts 25 msec before the beginning of the QRS complex and ends 125 msec after the end of that complex. This segment was subdivided into 24 overlapping subsegments in steps of 2 msec. The duration of each of these subsegments was then multiplied point-by-point by use of a window (Blackmann-Harris), and on each of these segments a 64-point fast Fourier transform was applied, covering the entire QRS complex. Four statistical variables, as defined by Kelen et al.,[23] were used for quantitative evaluation of the spectral turbulence analysis, applied on the average of the X, Y, and Z leads. With this analysis, the SAECG result was considered to be abnormal if three or more of the following variables were present: interslice correlation mean less than 92, interslice correlation standard deviation greater than 105, low slice correlation ratio greater than 73, and spectral entropy greater than 14. All spectral turbulence analysis measurements were obtained automatically.

Three methods of analysis were used with the signals obtained by the magnitude vector. The averaged ECG signals of the 61 patients with a narrow QRS were evaluated in time domain, and signals of the 23 patients with bundle branch block were assessed by frequency domain analysis.[8,16] The results from both subgroups were then combined (method 1). In the second step, the SAECG values in all patients were analyzed by the frequency domain technique (method 2). Finally, spectral turbulence analysis was applied to the SAECG in all patients (method 3). Abnormal criteria in any of the three methods used were considered pathologic findings.

Prevalence of SAECG Abnormalities

Abnormal values on SAECG were found in 62% of the patients (52 of 84) and in 17% of the healthy volunteers by at least one of the methods. The prevalence of SAECG abnormalities was always significantly lower in healthy volunteers (overall and for each of the methods) than in patients with Chagas' disease. Although patients in group A did not have obvious cardiac involvement, the prevalence of abnormal findings on SAECG (time domain, method 1; frequency domain, method 2) in these patients was higher than in the control group, but it was always lower than in patients with known cardiac damage (groups B, C, and D) (Fig. 6-3). No significant differences were observed in the prevalence of abnormal SAECG findings among subgroups B, C, and D with methods 1 and 2. However, when spectral turbulence analysis (method 3) was used, the patients in groups B and D (with electrical disturbance) had a higher prevalence of SAECG abnormalities than those in groups A and C.

Abnormal SAECG findings in the subgroup of asymptomatic patients (group A) might indicate early cardiac compromise. Andrade[4] reported finding myocardial fibrosis foci or autonomic denervation in seropositive patients without evidence of ECG changes. Similar findings have been reported after endomyocardial biopsy or in anatomicopathologic studies.[24,25] Pereira Barretto et al.[24] analyzed the biopsy specimens from 42 patients with Chagas' disease and demonstrated that only 31% of the asymptomatic patients with no ECG changes and normal chest radiograph had normal findings on biopsy. In this group

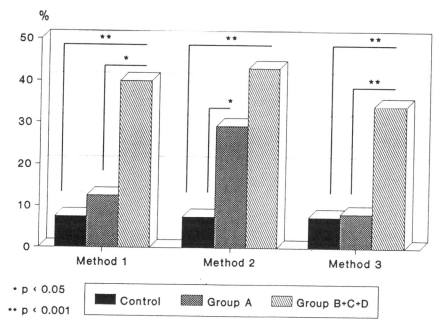

Fig. 6-3. Prevalence of abnormal signal-averaged electrocardiography findings in the control group, in patients without cardiac involvement (group A), and in patients with known cardiac damage (groups B, C, and D).

of patients, 12.5% had interstitial fibrosis, 50% myofibrillar degeneration, and 31.2% hypertrophy of cardiac fibers. The anatomicopathologic findings are very valuable if one takes into account that from an asymptomatic phase of the illness, cardiac compromise is already present. Abnormal SAECG findings in these patients support the hypothesis of early compromise of the myocardium, and this method could be a harmless and easy way to diagnose and predict this kind of myocardial compromise in patients in the early stages of the illness. This might explain the higher prevalence of abnormal SAECG findings in asymptomatic patients with Chagas' disease than in a control group. However, the only method that demonstrated statistically significant differences between these two cohorts was the analysis of SAECG by frequency domain (Fig. 6-3).

There was a correlation between abnormal SAECG findings and frequent and repetitive arrhythmias on the Holter recording (any method, $P < 0.05$; method 1, not significant; method 2, $P < 0.01$; method 3, $P < 0.004$) but not with ventricular dysfunction (Table 6-2).

Patients with abnormal SAECG results had worse ventricular function than those with normal results. However, the functional NYHA class, the cardiothoracic index, and the ejection fraction did not have a statistically significant influence on the prevalence of abnormalities on SAECG or the outcome. Gomes et al.[10] described a similar situation in 110 patients after acute myocardial infarction. They observed that those with abnormal SAECG findings had an ejection fraction similar to that of patients with normal findings.

In the present study, the prevalence of abnormal SAECG results was high, similar to that in patients who have had an acute myocardial infarction (30% to 40%), depending on the method used. It was, in turn, significantly higher than that in the healthy control group. De Moraes et al.[13] analyzed abnormal SAECG findings in patients with Chagas' disease and noted a prevalence of between 78% and 48%, corresponding principally to patients with sustained ventricular tachycardia at the beginning of the study. The results of de Moraes et al. are not comparable with those of our study because of differences in the classification and analysis of patients and because SAECG was

Table 6-2.

Correlation of Abnormal SAECG Findings,
Ventricular Dysfunction, and Complex Arrhythmia*

| Method | Ventricular dysfunction | | Complex arrhythmia | | | |
	RC	P	RC	P	OR	CI
1	0.718 ± 0.51	NS	0.451 ± 0.31	NS		
2	0.206 ± 0.50	NS	0.761 ± 0.31	<0.01	2.14	1.15–3.97
3	0.131 ± 0.56	NS	0.972 ± 0.32	<0.004	2.64	1.39–5.00

CI, 95% confidence interval; OR, odds ratio; RC, regression coefficient.
*Multivariate analysis (logistic regression).

done only with time domain. However, both studies agree in the finding of a high prevalence of abnormal SAECG results in this group of patients with Chagas' disease.

Predictors of Arrhythmic Events

Seventy-seven patients (92%) had follow-up during 30 months. One patient died from rupture of an abdominal aortic aneurysm and had normal SAECG findings in the baseline study. Eight of the 76 patients (10.5%) had serious arrhythmic events. All these patients belonged to groups B and D. Therefore, the actual prevalence of arrhythmic events in this subgroup of patients was higher, reaching 17.4%. Seven patients had sustained ventricular tachycardia, and one patient experienced sudden death. Seven of these eight patients had abnormal SAECG findings with at least one of the methods (four with method 1, seven with method 2, and three with method 3). Only one patient with normal SAECG findings had arrhythmic events (ventricular tachycardia) (2.2%). In contrast, the percentage of patients with abnormal SAECG results who had arrhythmic events was 22.5% ($P < 0.01$). The complex arrhythmic event survival rate (method of Kaplan-Meier) is shown in Figure 6 4. Thus, analysis of the absence and presence of abnormal SAECG findings in this population showed a sensitivity of 87.5%, a specificity of 58%, a positive predictive value of 22.5%, and a negative predictive value of 97.8% (method 2). These values are similar to those published previously in prospective studies of patients with coronary artery disease. Thus, although normal values are lacking in patients with Chagas' disease, analysis of SAECG seems to be a promising means of stratification in patients at risk for sustained ventricular tachyarrhythmias.

None of the asymptomatic patients in group A and none of the patients in group C had lethal arrhythmic events during follow-up.

De Moraes et al.[13] reported that the sensitivity and specificity of the abnormal SAECG results in patients with Chagas' disease with or without spontaneous sustained ventricular tachycardia were between 66% and 78% and 52% and 70%, respectively, depending on whether right bundle branch block was present.

Univariate analysis showed that the occurrence of malignant arrhythmic events was related to conduction disturbances ($P = 0.05$), frequent and repetitive ventricular premature contractions in the Holter recordings ($P < 0.003$), and abnormal SAECG findings detected by frequency domain analysis ($P < 0.007$). On the other hand, arrhythmic events were not correlated with either ventricular function or age.

The frequency domain analysis method was the most powerful independent predictor of malignant arrhythmic events. Cox regression analysis showed that the independent predictors of arrhythmic events were conduction disturbances ($P < 0.04$), frequent and repetitive arrhythmias on the Holter recording ($P < 0.03$), and abnormal SAECG

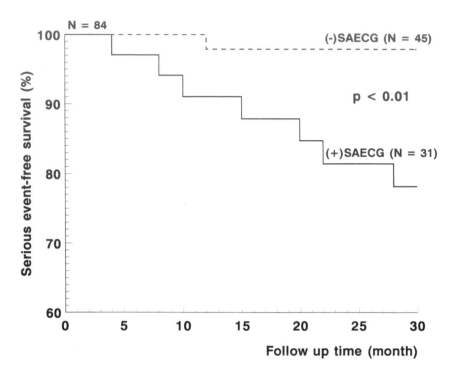

Fig. 6-4. Rate of 30-month serious event-free survival (Kaplan-Meier method). Of the original 84 patients, 8 were lost to follow-up. *Dashed line* and *continuous line* represent the 45 patients with normal and the 31 patients with abnormal signal-averaged electrocardiography (SAECG) findings, respectively ($P < 0.01$). The percentage of patients lost to follow-up was 10% in each group.

results by frequency domain analysis ($P < 0.05$) (Table 6-3). The last-named was the most powerful predictor (odds ratio, 11.7; 95% confidence interval, 3.13 to 36.6).

In contrast to findings in previous postinfarction studies,[26] adding the results of the time domain technique and spectral turbulence analy-

Table 6-3.
Independent Predictors of Malignant Arrhythmic Events*

	OR	CI	P
IVCD	10.5	1.16–93.7	<0.039
VPC	4.47	1.21–15.9	<0.027
SAECG abnormalities (method 2)	11.7	3.13–36.6	<0.042

CI, 95% confidence interval; IVCD, intraventricular conduction disturbances; OR, odds ratio; SAECG, signal-averaged electrocardiography; VPC, ventricular premature contractions.
*Multivariate analysis (logistic regression).

sis to those of the frequency analysis did not increase the predictive accuracy in our patients with Chagas' disease. However, the predictive value of signal averaging, especially with frequency domain analysis, remains controversial.[27,28]

The belief that the frequency domain method is the best predictor is controversial.[27,28] Kulakowski et al.[28] presented data in which this method did not help identify ventricular tachycardia in patients after myocardial infarction. The time domain method is always the most predictive. Nevertheless, Cain et al.[27] showed that the frequency domain provided better differentiation than the time domain between patients with and those without ventricular tachycardia. In their work, 91% of the patients were correctly identified by frequency domain compared with 70% by time domain. They concluded that because the variables for the frequency domain are not standardized, the discrepancies arise from signal processing problems and the definition of areas. In Chagas' disease, no standardized criteria exist for either of the analytical methods. In our work, different areas were analyzed and the processing was done under the guidelines described by Cain et al.[27]

Arrhythmogenic Substrate

The origin of abnormal findings on SAECG has been attributed to a slow and fragmented conduction area large enough to be recorded from the surface of the body.[7,8] In patients with myocardial infarction, the transition area located between the viable cardiac muscle and the necrotic or fibrotic tissue is considered the basis for the reentrant mechanism during ventricular tachycardia and the origin of abnormal SAECG findings.[7,8] The mechanism leading to the occurrence of SAECG abnormalities in Chagas' disease has not yet been established. However, some alternatives might be hypothesized. First, the involvement of coronary microvasculature could produce multiple areas of fibrosis, in turn causing multiple potential reentrant circuits.[23,25] These areas must be large enough to be recorded from the body surface and must have determined electrophysiologic characteristics to allow reentry. This theory would explain false-negative and false-positive findings in SAECG from the body surface. Second, abnormal SAECG findings might originate from the limits of ventricular aneurysms[29] that allow macroreentrant circuits. Bestetti et al.[30] and de Paola et al.[5] suggested the importance of ventricular aneurysms as an anatomical substrate for the development of sustained ventricular arrhythmias and sudden death in patients with Chagas' disease.

The inducibility of sustained ventricular tachycardia during programmed ventricular stimulation suggests a reentrant mechanism for arrhythmia. However, the role of this technique in patients with Chagas' disease seems to be of controversial clinical interest. This affirmation is based on published data demonstrating that in patients with spontaneous episodes of ventricular tachycardia, the inducibility of this arrhythmia ranges from 40% to 100%.[14,31] This finding reaffirms the need of noninvasive diagnostic tools for risk stratification in these patients.

Conclusions

1. Abnormal SAECG findings are frequent in patients with Chagas' disease.
2. Abnormal SAECG tracings are associated with frequent and complex ventricular arrhythmias.
3. Frequent ventricular arrhythmias during baseline Holter recording, intraventricular conduction disturbances in the surface ECG, and abnormal SAECG results by frequency domain analysis are independent predictors of developing malignant arrhythmic events (sustained ventricular tachycardia or sudden death or both).

Acknowledgments: We thank colleagues who collaborated in different stages of this work: Josep Guindo, M.D., Wojciech Zareba, M.D., Xavier Viñolas, M.D., Mario I. Cámera, M.D., Branco Mautner, M.D., Antonio Bayés de Luna, M.D., and Jose Tessler, M.D. We also thank Mr. Etienne van Dam for his help in preparing this manuscript.

References

1. World Health Organization: Sixth programme report. Chapter 6: Chagas' disease. UNDP, World Bank, WHO. Special programme for research and training in tropical disease. Document TDR,PR-6,83.6-CHA, 1983
2. Hagar JM, Rahimtoola SH: Chagas' heart disease in the United States. N Engl J Med 325:763-768, 1991
3. Rosenbaum MB: Chagasic myocardiopathy. Prog Cardiovasc Dis 7:199-225, 1964
4. Andrade ZA: Mechanisms of myocardial damage in *Trypanosoma cruzi* infection. *In* Cytopathology of Parasitic Disease (Ciba Foundation Symposium 99). Edited by D Evered, GM Collins. London, Pitman Books, 1983, p 214
5. de Paola AA, Horowitz LN, Miyamoto MH, Pinheiro R, Ferreira DF, Terzian AB, Cirenza C, Guiguer N Jr, Portugal OP: Angiographic and electrophysiologic substrates of ventricular tachycardia in chronic Chagasic myocarditis. Am J Cardiol 65:360-363, 1990
6. Manzullo EC: Epidemiología de la Enfermedad de Chagas en la Argentina. Rev Fed Arg Cardiol 17:141, 1988
7. Simson MB: Use of signals in the terminal QRS complex to identify patients with ventricular tachycardia after myocardial infarction. Circulation 64:235-242, 1981
8. Breithardt G, Cain ME, el-Sherif N, Flowers N, Hombach V, Janse M, Simson MB, Steinbeck G: Standards for analysis of ventricular late potentials using high resolution or signal-averaged electrocardiography. A statement by a Task Force Committee between the European Society of Cardiol-

ogy, the American Heart Association and the American College of Cardiology. Eur Heart J 12:473-480, 1991

9. Steinberg JS, Regan A, Sciacca RR, Bigger JT Jr, Fleiss JL: Predicting arrhythmic events after acute myocardial infarction using the signal-averaged electrocardiogram. Am J Cardiol 69:13-21, 1992

10. Gomes JA, Winters SL, Martinson M, Machac J, Stewart D, Targonski A: The prognostic significance of quantitative signal-averaged variables relative to clinical variables, site of myocardial infarction, ejection fraction and ventricular premature beats: a prospective study. J Am Coll Cardiol 13:377-384, 1989

11. Guindo J, Madoery C, Esparza E, Viñolas X, Zareba W, Martinez Rubio A, Mautner B, Madoery R, Breithardt G, Bayés de Luna A: Cardiac involvement in Chagas' disease: arrhythmic profile. In The New Frontiers of Arrhythmias, 1992, pp 505-512

12. Madoery C, Guindo J, Esparza E, Viñolas X, Zareba W, Martinez A, Mautner B, Madoery R, Breithardt G, Bayés de Luna A: ECG de señal promediada en la enfermedad de Chagas. Rev Arg Cardiol 60:93-102, 1992

13. de Moraes AP, Moffa PJ, Sosa EA, Bellotti GM, Pastore CA, Lima EV, Chalela WA, Grupi CJ, Pileggi FJ: Signal-averaged electrocardiogram in chronic Chagas' heart disease. Rev Paul Med 113:851-857, 1995

14. Giniger AG, Retyk EO, Laino RA, Sananes EG, Lapuente AR: Ventricular tachycardia in Chagas' disease. Am J Cardiol 70:459-462, 1992

15. Kienzle MG, Miller J, Falcone RA, Harken A, Josephson ME: Intraoperative endocardial mapping during sinus rhythm: relationship to site of origin of ventricular tachycardia. Circulation 70:957-965, 1984

16. Cain ME, Ambos HD, Witkowski FX, Sobel BE: Fast-Fourier transform analysis of signal-averaged electrocardiograms for identification of patients prone to sustained ventricular tachycardia. Circulation 69:711-720, 1984

17. Zareba W, Guindo J, Madoery C, Viñolas X, Torner P, Oter R, Bayés de Luna A: Late potentials diagnosing by FFT frequency analysis in patients with bundle branch block—comparison of different area ratios (abstract). Eur Heart J 12 Suppl D:12, 1991

18. Poll DS, Marchlinski FE, Falcone RA, Josephson ME, Simson MB: Abnormal signal-averaged electrocardiograms in patients with nonischemic congestive cardiomyopathy: relationship to sustained ventricular tachyarrhythmias. Circulation 72:1308-1313, 1985

19. Middlekauff HR, Stevenson WG, Woo MA, Moser DK, Stevenson LW: Comparison of frequency of late potentials in idiopathic dilated cardiomyopathy and ischemic cardiomyopathy with advanced congestive heart failure and their usefulness in predicting sudden death. Am J Cardiol 66:1113-1117, 1990

20. Signal-averaged electrocardiography. J Am Coll Cardiol 27:238-249, 1996

21. Madoery C, Guindo J, Esparza E, Viñolas X, Zareba W, Martinez A, Mautner B, Madoery R, Breithardt G, Bayes de Luna A: Signal-averaged ECG in Chagas disease: incidence of late potentials and relationship to cardiac involvement (abstract). J Am Coll Cardiol 19 Suppl:324A, 1992

22. Araujo FG, Chiari E, Dias JC: Demonstration of Trypanosoma cruzi antigen in serum from patients with Chagas' disease. Lancet 1:246-249, 1981

23. Kelen GJ, Henkin R, Starr AM, Caref EB, Bloomfield D, el-Sherif N: Spectral turbulence analysis of the signal-averaged electrocardiogram and its

predictive accuracy for inducible sustained monomorphic ventricular tachycardia. Am J Cardiol 67:965-975, 1991

24. Pereira Barretto AC, Mady C, Arteaga-Fernandez E, Stolf N, Lopes EA, Higuchi ML, Bellotti G, Pileggi F: Right ventricular endomyocardial biopsy in chronic Chagas' disease. Am Heart J 111:307-312, 1986

25. Rossi MA, Goncalves S, Ribeiro-dos-Santos R: Experimental *Trypanosoma cruzi* cardiomyopathy in BALB/c mice. The potential role of intravascular platelet aggregation in its genesis. Am J Pathol 114:209-216, 1984

26. Ahuja RK, Turitto G, Ibrahim B, Caref EB, el-Sherif N: Combined time-domain and spectral turbulence analysis of the signal-averaged ECG improves its predictive accuracy in postinfarction patients. J Electrocardiol 27 Suppl:202-206, 1994

27. Cain ME, Lindsay BD, Arthur RM, Markham J, Ambos HD: Noninvasive detection of patients prone to life-threatening ventricular arrhythmias by frequency analysis of electrocardiographic signals. *In* Cardiac Electrophysiology: From Cell to Bedside. Edited by DP Zipes, J Jalife. Philadelphia, WB Saunders Company, 1990, pp 817-830

28. Kulakowski P, Malik M, Poloniecki J, Bashir Y, Odemuyiwa O, Farrell T, Staunton A, Camm J: Frequency versus time domain analysis of signal-averaged electrocardiograms. II. Identification of patients with ventricular tachycardia after myocardial infarction. J Am Coll Cardiol 20:135-143, 1992

29. Oliveira JS, Mello De Oliveira JA, Frederigue U Jr, Lima Filho EC: Apical aneurysm of Chagas's heart disease. Br Heart J 46:432-437, 1981

30. Bestetti RB, Santos CR, Machado-Junior OB, Ariolli MT, Carmo JL, Costa NK, de Oliveira RB: Clinical profile of patients with Chagas' disease before and during sustained ventricular tachycardia. Int J Cardiol 29:39-46, 1990

31. Boccardo D, Tibaldi M, Coll M, Conci E, Serra C: Estimulación ventricula programada en la evaluación de pacientes chagásicos con arritmia ventricular. *In* Actualizaciones en la Enfermedad de Chagas. Edited by RJ Madoery, C Madoery, MI Cámera. Buenos Aires, Organismo Oficial del Congreso Nacional de Medicina, 1993, pp 163

Chapter 7

Clinical Relevance of Invasive Electrophysiologic Studies in Patients with Chagas' Disease

Cidio Halperin, M.D., Sérgio Rassi, M.D.

Cardiac Chagas' disease is classically characterized by the manifestation of three clinical syndromes: congestive heart failure, thromboembolic disease, and arrhythmogenic disturbance. They may occur together or independently, in different levels of cardiac involvement.[1]

As in any idiopathic cardiomyopathy, arrhythmias in this endemic tropical disease can range from atrial ectopic beats to cardiac arrest, with no relationship to left ventricular function.[2] It is said that in Chagas' disease, we may find an "encyclopedia" of disorders of the cardiac rhythm.[3]

Comprehensive use of noninvasive diagnostic tools should always precede an invasive electrophysiologic study (EPS). These approaches are discussed in detail elsewhere in this book.[4,5]

The rest electrocardiogram, Holter monitoring, stress exercise test, loop recording, and tilt table testing are of fundamental importance in achieving an accurate diagnosis,[6] but if noninvasive procedures fail to be diagnostic, an invasive approach may be used.

Because paroxysms ("storms") in the occurrence of arrhythmias are likely, patients may have apparently normal test results, so that different ways of evaluating nonspontaneous arrhythmias may be necessary.[3]

The diagnostic EPS requires venipunctures and the positioning of multiple multipolar catheters, usually in the high right atria, the tricuspid annulus (His bundle electrogram recording), and at least one site

From Tentori MC, Segura EL, Hayes DL (eds.) *Arrhythmia Management in Chagas' Disease*. Armonk, NY: Futura Publishing Co., Inc. ©2000.

in the right ventricle. Myocardial regional electrical activity is recorded and conduction intervals are measured, and programmed electrical (atrial or ventricular) stimulation may be used to evaluate tissue refractoriness and to induce or terminate arrhythmia, with or without drug sensitization.

The EPS may be quite useful in patients with unexplained syncope, atrioventricular (AV) or intraventricular block, sinus node dysfunction, or tachyarrhythmias.[3,7-10]

In the chagasic population, the main cause of syncope is ventricular tachycardia (36%), followed by severe damage to the His-Purkinje system (25%) and sick sinus syndrome (14%).[8]

Electrophysiologic Study in Bradyarrhythmias

In Chagas' disease, a diffuse lesion of the myocardium is usual[11] and an exclusive disturbance of the conduction system itself is rare. In addition, bradyarrhythmias and tachyarrhythmias are frequently associated.[12]

Among 155 patients with Chagas' disease and clinical evidence of sick sinus syndrome, the electrophysiologic findings in 38% showed the characteristic form of bradycardia-tachycardia syndrome (Fig. 7-1) and in 70.5% induction of some kind of sustained supraventricular tachyarrhythmia, usually uncommon atrial flutter or atrial fibrillation, especially in those with ventricular dysfunction. During programmed electrical stimulation of the right ventricle, with up to three extrastimuli, 17% of the patients with sick sinus syndrome also had induction of sustained ventricular tachycardia.[13] Simultaneous alteration of the AV node properties was found in 47% of the patients.[8] Multiple AV nodal pathways have been reported, but the clinical significance of this finding remains to be determined.[14]

AV dysfunction may be clinically manifested by different degrees of AV block.[7] At electrophysiologic evaluation of chagasic patients with AV conduction disturbances, 20% had compromised infra-Hisian structures (basal HV interval > 70 msec; HV block with atrial pacing at cycle length > 500 msec) (Fig. 7-2).

First-degree AV block usually originates from the AV node, but with a wide QRS complex, it may occur at the proximal His-Purkinje system and compromise the prognosis. More rarely, a narrow QRS complex associated with first-degree AV block may also be associated with infra-Hisian damage (Fig. 7-3). Bifascicular bundle branch block with AV node delay may also account for the first-degree block.

Second-degree block (Mobitz type I) may in the same way have its origin at the AV node (more common) or in the His-Purkinje system (Fig. 7-4). We observed that this type of block occurring during an exercise stress test usually is associated with a dysfunction in the His-Purkinje system (proximal or distal).

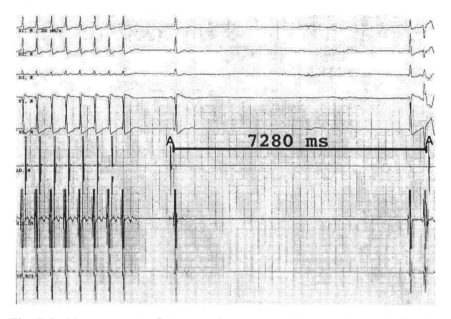

Fig. 7-1. Measurement of sinus node recovery time (pacing cycle length, 400 msec) in a patient with sinus node arrest of 2 seconds on Holter monitoring and symptoms of near-syncope. The measured atrial pause was 7,280 msec, and the corrected sinus node recovery time was 5,890 msec. The tracing sequence is, from the top, leads I, II, III, V_1, V_6, HRA (high right atrium), HB (His bundle), and RVA (right ventricular apex). The recording speed was 25 mm/sec.

Complete AV block (Fig. 7-5) is not unusual in chagasic cardiomyopathy, whereas it may be an occasional finding in an asymptomatic or even classic Stokes-Adams syndrome.

The so-called pathognomonic electrocardiographic presentation of Chagas' disease is an intraventricular conduction abnormality: right bundle branch block with left anterior-superior fascicular block.

In an evaluation of the conduction system during EPS in 304 patients with intraventricular branch block and clinical manifestations of syncope or near-syncope, different levels of commitment of the conduction system were demonstrated (Table 7-1).

In patients with chagasic cardiomyopathy and bradyarrhythmias, invasive EPS may be useful in the evaluation of the sinus node and conduction system, especially in patients with unexplained syncope or near-syncope.[9] In sick sinus syndrome, detection of atrial tachyarrhythmias or diffuse conduction tissue disease is certainly a determinant factor when pacemaker therapy is considered, with or without adjunctive drug therapy.[15,16]

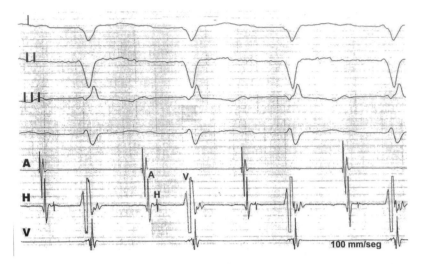

Fig. 7-2. Baseline electrophysiologic tracing from a patient in sinus rhythm who had right bundle branch block with left axis deviation shows long HV interval (200 msec) during 1:1 atrioventricular conduction. The tracing sequence is, from the top, leads I, II, III, V₁, HRA (high right atrium), HB (His bundle), and RVA (right ventricular apex). The recording speed was 25 mm/sec.

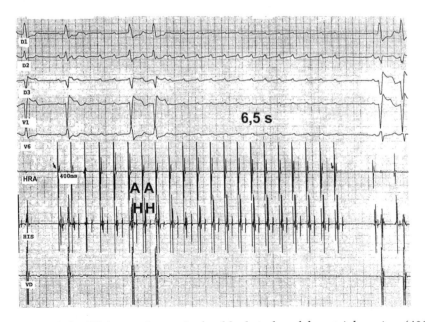

Fig. 7-3. Infra-Hisian atrioventricular block induced by atrial pacing (400 msec) with ventricular asystole of 6.5 seconds. The tracing sequence is, from the top, leads I, II, III, V₁, V₆, HRA (high right atrium), HB (His bundle), and RVA (right ventricular apex).

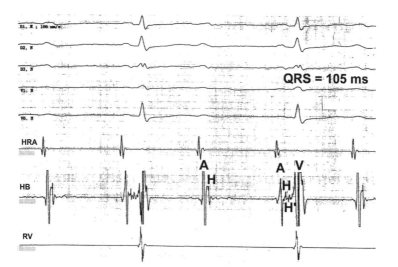

Fig. 7-4. 2:1 Atrioventricular block with narrow QRS complex and intra-Hisian block (H-H'). The tracing sequence is, from the top, leads I, II, III, V₁, V₆, HRA (high right atrium), HB (His bundle), and RVA (right ventricular apex). The recording speed was 100 mm/sec.

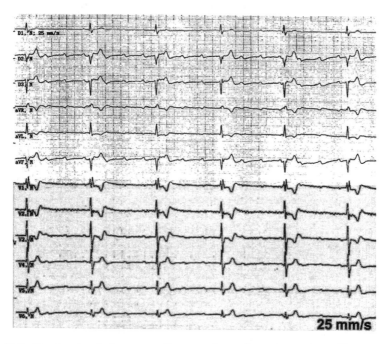

Fig. 7-5. Twelve-lead electrocardiogram in a chagasic patient. Heart rate is 36 bpm with complete atrioventricular block and QRS configuration of right bundle branch block and left anterior hemiblock.

Table 7-1.

Relationship Between Electrocardiographic Presentation of Intraventricular Branch Block and Intra- or Infra-Hisian Compromise at Electrophysiologic Study in Patients with Chagas' Disease

ECG	RBBB, %	LBBB, %	RBBB + LAH %	RBBB + LPH, %	RBBB + LAH + 1° AVB, %
Infra-Hisian involvement	12	52	19	33	44

1° AVB, first-degree atrioventricular block; ECG, electrocardiogram; LAH, left anterior hemiblock; LBBB, left bundle branch block; LPH, left posterior hemiblock; RBBB, right bundle branch block.

Electrophysiologic Study in Tachyarrhythmias

Paroxysmal sustained ventricular tachyarrhythmia is possibly the major problem in chagasic cardiomyopathy. Because of high rates of morbidity and mortality, this disorder is a highly significant public health issue, particularly in patients with ventricular dysfunction.[17,18]

In 91% of patients with clinically documented ventricular tachycardia, EPS with standard programmed ventricular stimulation protocol successfully reproduced the anomaly, with up to three extrastimuli in the right ventricular apex (85%) or in the outflow tract (15%).[3]

The QRS morphology during ventricular tachycardia usually has a right bundle branch block pattern with superior (45%) (Fig. 7-6) or inferior (32%) axis deviation.[3]

The presumed mechanism is a macroreentrant circuit, in some cases with intramyocardial or epicardial components.[19,20] Scanning electron microscopic studies have demonstrated diffuse myocardial disease with scars and inflammatory fibrosis,[11] an indication for some investigators to use alternative radioisotopic mapping techniques.[21] The inferior basal septal region[13] of the left ventricle seems to be the most frequent site of the reentry circuit (Fig. 7-7 and 7-8), although the lateral and the posterobasal septal sites have also been described.[17,19]

EPS may be used to establish the therapeutic efficacy of antiarrhythmic drugs in patients with sustained ventricular tachycardia.[3,10,13] A class III antiarrhythmic drug, amiodarone,[4,5,9-11,17,19,20] has been shown to decrease the total and arrhythmic mortality. A similar benefit has been reported in patients with clinically documented ventricular arrhythmias and empirical use of amiodarone.[22] These trials suggest that the incidence of the drug side effects is limited.[10,17,22]

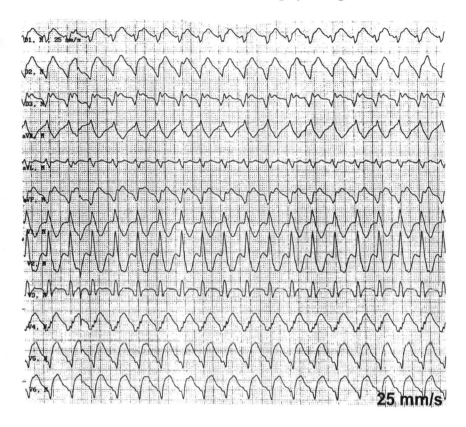

Fig. 7-6. Sustained monomorphic ventricular tachycardia with right bundle branch block morphology and left axis deviation (12-lead electrocardiogram).

Catheter ablation procedures using radio frequency as the energy source have been reported as alternative therapy for sustained ventricular tachyarrhythmias (Chapter 9). The extensive myocardial involvement in Chagas' disease may be responsible for the lack of efficacy of the usual forms of endocardial mapping. The eventual appearance of not only subendocardial but also transmural or even epicardial arrhythmia circuits was the rationale for the development of alternative myocardial mapping techniques.[12,13]

Only a few preliminary reports have appeared on the use of the implantable cardioverter-defibrillator in patients with Chagas' disease and malignant ventricular arrhythmias.[23,24] Periods with an increased incidence of ventricular arrhythmias (so-called arrhythmic storms) may indicate that adjunctive nonpharmacologic therapy is needed.[4,5,9-11,14,18,20-22,25,26]

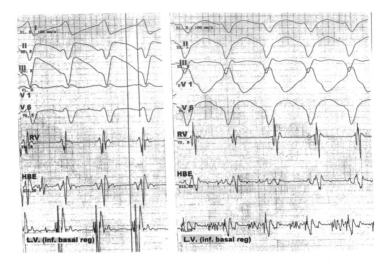

Fig. 7-7. Endocardial electrophysiologic mapping during ventricular tachycardia induced in the laboratory. In the two different morphologic types, the earliest "V" potential (–95 msec) in the inferobasal portion of the left ventricle is associated with fractionated diastolic potentials. The tracing sequence is, from the top, leads I, II, III, V_1, V_6, RVA (right ventricular apex), HB (His bundle), and VE (exploring catheter positioned in the inferobasal area of the left ventricle). The recording speed was 100 mm/sec.

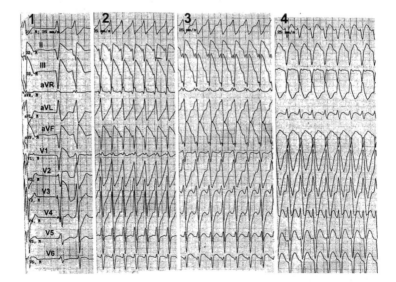

Fig. 7-8. Twelve-lead electrocardiographic tracings from the patient in Figure 7-7. Three different morphologic types (tracings 2, 3, and 4) of sustained ventricular tachycardia are shown. Tracing 1 is the baseline rhythm. A permanent pacemaker was previously implanted because of severe bradyarrhythmia.

Conclusion

Arrhythmogenic cardiac involvement in Chagas' disease may be signaled by a myriad of abnormal findings. The potential direct (immunologic) or indirect (inflammatory) involvement of any structure of the conduction system may be the agent for bradyarrhythmias and tachyarrhythmias.[11] The invasive EPS may be valuable in evaluating syncope, selecting therapy for ventricular tachyarrhythmias, and clarifying abnormal patterns of AV conduction in patients with Chagas' disease.

References

1. Rassi A, Rassi SG, Rassi A Jr: Chagas disease: clinical features. In Chagas Disease (American Trypanosomiasis): Its Impact on Transfusion and Clinical Medicine. Edited by S Wendel, Z Brenes. São Paulo, 1992, pp 81-101
2. Rassi A, Lorga AM, Rassi SG: Diagnose and treatment of arrhythmias on chronic cardiopathy. In Chagas Cardiopathy. Edited by JR Cançado, M Chuster. Belo Horizonte, Imprensa Oficial do Estado de Minas Gerais, 1985, pp 274-288
3. Rassi SG: Electrophysiology study on chagasic chronic miocardites. The Brazilian Society of Tropical Medicine 26 Suppl 11, 1993
4. de Paola AA, Gomes JA, Terzian AB, Miyamoto MH, Martinez Fo EE: Ventricular tachycardia during exercise testing as a predictor of sudden death in patients with chronic chagasic cardiomyopathy and ventricular arrhythmias. Br Heart J 74:293-295, 1995
5. Grupi CJ, Moffa PJ, Barbosa SA, Sanches PC, Barragan Filho EG, Bellotti GM, Pileggi FJ: Holter monitoring in Chagas' heart disease. Rev Paul Med 113:835-840, 1995
6. Rassi A, Rassi A Jr, Rassi AG, et al: Chronic cardiopathy—arrhythmias. In Clínica e Terapêutica da Doença de Chagas. Uma Abordagem Prática Para O Clínico Geral. Edited by JCP Dias, JR E Coura. Rio de Janeiro, Fio Cruz, 1997, pp 201-222
7. Rassi SG: Átrio-ventricular blocks. Bulletin of the Arrhythmia and Electrophysiology Department of the Brazilian Society of Cardiology, No. 1, January 1990
8. Rassi SG, Pimenta J: Electrophysiologic evaluation of brady-arrhythmias. In Eletrofisiologia Clínica e Intervensionista das Arritmias Cardíacas. Edited by FES Cruz, IG F.° E Maia. Rio de Janeiro, Reventes Ltda, 1997, pp 91-106
9. Martinelli Filho M, Sosa E, Nishioka S, Scanavacca M, Bellotti G, Pileggi F: Clinical and electrophysiologic features of syncope in chronic chagasic heart disease. J Cardiovasc Electrophysiol 5:563-570, 1994
10. Giniger AG, Retyk EO, Laino RA, Sananes EG, Lapuente AR: Ventricular tachycardia in Chagas' disease. Am J Cardiol 70:459-462, 1992
11. Rossi MA: Fibrosis and inflammatory cells in human chronic chagasic myocarditis: scanning electron microscopy and immunohistochemical observations. Int J Cardiol 66:183-194, 1998

12. Rassi A, Lorga AM, Rassi SG: Diagnostic and therapeutic approach of the chronic Chagas-related cardiopathy. *In* Diagnosis and Treatment of Cardiac Arrhythmias. Third edition. Edited by H Germiniani. Rio de Janeiro, Guanabara Koogan S. A., 1990, pp 225-244

13. Rassi Junior A, Gabriel Rassi A, Gabriel Rassi S, Rassi Junior L, Rassi A: Ventricular arrhythmia in Chagas disease. Diagnostic, prognostic, and therapeutic features [Portuguese]. Arq Bras Cardiol 65:377-387, 1995

14. Pimenta J, Miranda M, Silva LA: Abnormal atrioventricular nodal response patterns in patients with long-term Chagas' disease. Chest 78:310-315, 1980

15. Sosa EA, Lorga AM, Paola AA, Maia IG, Pimenta J, Gizzi JC, Rassi SG: Indications for intracardiac electrophysiological studies—1988. Recommendations of the Committee of the Society of Cardiology of the State of Sao Paulo and of the Arrhythmia and Electrophysiology Study Group of the Brazilian Society of Cardiology [Portuguese]. Arq Bras Cardiol 51:427-428, 1988

16. Lorga AM, de Paola AA, Sosa EA, Maia IG, Pimenta J, Gizzi JC, Rassi SG: Selection of the mode of definitive artificial cardiac stimulation. Recommendations of the Committee of Arrhythmia and Electrophysiology Study Groups of the Brazilian Society of Cardiology [Portuguese]. Arq Bras Cardiol 51:287-288, 1988

17. Doval HC, Nul DR, Grancelli HO, Perrone SV, Bortman GR, Curiel R for Grupo de Estudio de la Sobrevida en la Insuficiencia Cardiaca en Argentina: Randomised trial of low-dose amiodarone in severe congestive heart failure. Lancet 344:493-498, 1994

18. Barretto AC, Mady C, Ianni BM, Arteaga E, Cardoso RH, da Luz PL, Pileggi F: Relationship between ventricular arrhythmia and cardiac function in Chagas disease [Portuguese]. Arq Bras Cardiol 64:533-535, 1995

19. de Paola AAV, Melo WDS, Távora MZP, Martinez EE: Angiographic and electrophysiological substrates for ventricular tachycardia mapping through the coronary veins. Heart 79:59-63, 1998

20. Sosa E, Scanavacca M, D'Avila A, Piccioni J, Sanchez O, Velarde JL, Silva M, Reolao B: Endocardial and epicardial ablation guided by nonsurgical transthoracic epicardial mapping to treat recurrent ventricular tachycardia. J Cardiovasc Electrophysiol 9:229-239, 1998

21. de Paola AA, Balbao CE, Castiglioni ML, Barbieri A, Mendonca A, Netto OS, Guiguer Junior N, Vattimo AC, Souza IA, Portugal OP, et al: Radioisotopic mapping of the arrhythmogenic focus in patients with chronic chagasic cardiomyopathy and sustained ventricular tachycardia [Portuguese]. Arq Bras Cardiol 60:373-376, 1993

22. Scanavacca MI, Sosa EA, Lee JH, Bellotti G, Pileggi F: Empiric therapy with amiodarone in patients with chronic Chagas cardiomyopathy and sustained ventricular tachycardia [Portuguese]. Arq Bras Cardiol 54:367-371, 1990

23. Trappe HJ, Fieguth HG, Klein H, Wenzlaff P, Weber-Conrad O, Schohl W, Kielblock B, Lichtlen PR: The importance of the underlying disease for outcome of patients with implanted automatic defibrillators [German]. Med Klin 88:362-370, 1993

24. Lessmeier TJ, Lehmann MH, Steinman RT, Fromm BS, Akhtar M, Calkins H, DiMarco JP, Epstein AE, Estes NA, Fogoros RN, Marchlinski FE, Wilber DJ: Outcome with implantable cardioverter-defibrillator therapy for survivors of ventricular fibrillation secondary to idiopathic dilated cardiomyop-

athy or coronary artery disease without myocardial infarction. Am J Cardiol 72:911-915, 1993

25. Pimenta J, de Souza C, Valente N: Long-term follow-up of patients with Chagas' heart disease and right bundle branch block. Comparative study with non-chagasic patients with bundle branch block (abstract). Pacing Clin Electrophysiol 17:843, 1994

26. Sternick EB, Sobrinho AL, Lisboa JC, Barbosa MR, Fantini F, Gontijo Filho B, Vrandecic MO: Transcoronary chemical ablation of ventricular tachycardia in a patient with chronic Chagas cardiomyopathy [Portuguese]. Arq Bras Cardiol 58:307-310, 1992

Chapter 8

Pharmacologic Treatment of Arrhythmias Related to Chronic Chagas' Heart Disease

Marcelo V. Elizari, M.D., F.A.C.C., F.A.H.A., Pablo A. Chiale, M.D.

Cardiac involvement in Chagas' disease is an important health problem in Latin American countries where the disease is endemic.[1] Most persons chronically infected with *Trypanosoma cruzi* (about 70%) never have any evidence of myocardial compromise, although the infection is lifelong. However, 15 to 20 years after the initial and usually unrecognized infection, up to 30% of those infected ultimately have symptoms or signs of visceral damage. Although digestive lesions and neurologic disorders are observed in some cases, the most important and frequent clinical manifestation is chronic cardiomyopathy.[2,3]

The pathogenesis of chronic Chagas' heart disease is partially understood, and several hypotheses have been formed. Many studies have proposed an outstanding role for immunologic disorders triggered by the parasite and the influence of autoimmune mechanisms.[4-8] The lack of correlation between the location and number of parasitized myocytes and the severity, type, and extension of the inflammatory lesions largely supports this assumption. Clinical and experimental studies have demonstrated that circulating antibodies directed against different components of *T. cruzi* may crossreact with autonomic membrane receptors of myocardial cells. Other mechanisms, such as microvascular dysfunction,[9] myocardial ischemia,[10] autonomic nervous system

From Tentori MC, Segura EL, Hayes DL (eds.) *Arrhythmia Management in Chagas' Disease.* Armonk, NY: Futura Publishing Co., Inc. ©2000.

[1]This paper was supported by Fundación de Investigaciones Cardiológicas Einthoven.

impairment,[11,12] and autoimmune and microvascular abnormalities,[13] have also been implicated.

In the most advanced forms of the disease, the cardiac pathologic findings are those of dilated cardiomyopathy, including biventricular and atrial dilatation, hypertrophy, diffuse active myocarditis, and fibrosis. In 1964, Rosenbaum[3] coined the term "panmyocarditis" to describe the histologic picture of the heart lesions, which are microfocal and disseminated throughout the heart. Confluent areas of fibrosis and apical aneurysms with thrombi are common and distinctive findings.[14]

The anatomicopathologic features of myocardial lesions and the "panmyocarditis" concept explain the wide spectrum of electrocardiographic (ECG) morphologic abnormalities and arrhythmias often found in the advanced forms of chronic chagasic cardiomyopathy (CChM). Atrial damage accounts for the variety of atrial bradyarrhythmias and tachyarrhythmias, and involvement of the ventricles sets the stage for atrioventricular and intraventricular conduction disturbances and for a number of ventricular arrhythmias.[2,3,15]

Progression of CChM leads to heart failure and sudden death. In a follow-up study in San Felipe, Brazil,[16] 58% of deaths in the chagasic population were the consequence of refractory cardiac failure and 37% were sudden deaths. In contrast, Reis Lopes et al.[17] reported that 17.6% of chagasic patients autopsied had experienced sudden death apparently without previous symptoms of cardiac disease. Although conclusive proof is not available, there is general agreement that ventricular fibrillation is the arrhythmia that precipitates sudden death.[3,16,17] In turn, sudden death can be heralded by complex ventricular arrhythmias.[18,19]

Ventricular premature contractions (VPCs) (and intraventricular conduction disturbances) are usually the earliest manifestations of ventricular involvement.[19] When ambulatory ECG monitoring is performed, VPCs can be detected in about 10% of infected persons with normal ECG findings and without other evidence of cardiac involvement. However, in patients with intraventricular conduction disturbances and abnormal ventriculographic findings (without clinical evidence of cardiac failure), the prevalence of VPCs increases to 56%. Moreover, virtually all patients with heart failure have frequent uniform or multiform ventricular premature beats and runs of nonsustained ventricular tachycardia.[19] In fact, a number of chagasic patients have ventricular arrhythmias resembling the "potentially malignant ventricular arrhythmias," and this implies an enhanced risk of sudden cardiac death, such as that described for ischemic heart disease.[20] Patients with these ventricular arrhythmias are subject to the development of symptoms (syncope or near-syncope), sustained and recurrent ventricular tachycardia, or ventricular fibrillation.[21-25] (Fig. 8-1). Since these arrhythmias are undoubtedly related to sudden cardiac death,[2,3,15-19,21-25] recognition and knowing the best approach to treatment are of paramount importance.

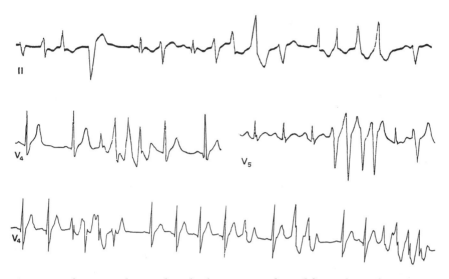

Fig. 8-1. Electrocardiographic rhythm strips selected from three chagasic patients with potentially malignant ventricular arrhythmias. Ventricular premature contractions are frequent, multiform, repetitive, and short-coupling, with R on T phenomenon.

This chapter essentially describes the main characteristics of the potentially malignant ventricular arrhythmias of CChM and, according to our experience, current pharmacologic treatment. A brief reference to the management of supraventricular arrhythmias is included.

Ventricular Arrhythmias

Potentially Malignant Ventricular Arrhythmias

In a previous report,[21] we described and analyzed the ECG characteristics of the ventricular arrhythmias in patients with severe CChM. In all patients, ventricular ectopy met at least two of the following criteria: multiformity, repetitiveness, and short coupling interval (R on T phenomenon). This highly selected group had the most complex ventricular arrhythmias; hence, the findings should not be extrapolated to chagasic patients with less serious ventricular arrhythmias. In this group of 28 patients, 203 conventional ECGs with rhythm strips lasting 1 to 5 minutes obtained at various intervals (3 to 30 days) during a 3-month period showed the abnormalities mentioned above in most of the tracings. Multiformity of ventricular extrasystoles was the most constant ECG finding (Fig. 8-1, top strip). This was observed even with a very low number of VPCs in most patients.

Ventricular parasystole is recognized in Holter recordings from many patients or, when looked for, in long ECG strips. Probably, CChM is the cardiopathy with the highest incidence of this arrhythmia.[15]

In another group of 41 patients with CChM who had potentially malignant ventricular arrhythmias,[26] 8 had recurrent syncope, 6 dizziness, 22 palpitations, and 11 cardiac failure. Thirty-three patients had myocardial enlargement, and 31 had intraventricular or atrioventricular conduction disturbances. Thus, these arrhythmias generally occur in association with moderate to severe myocardial damage, a relevant factor for the choice of the most convenient antiarrhythmic treatment.

Relationship of Autonomic Nervous System, Cardiac Rate, and Ventricular Arrhythmias

In about 60% of the patients with complex ventricular arrhythmias (couplets, multiformity, and R on T phenomenon), number and complexity are not significantly modified by rest or sleep, slight or moderate efforts, emotions, or corresponding changes in heart rate. The striking steadiness of ventricular arrhythmias indicates that the underlying electrophysiologic mechanism remains operative irrespective of the prevailing autonomic tone. On the contrary, in the remaining 40% of patients, the frequency and complexity of VPCs increase with emotional and physical stress and decrease during sleep or rest (Fig. 8-2). Concomitantly, heart rate increases and decreases, respectively. Again, regardless of the number and complexity of ventricular arrhythmias, multiformity remains unmodified.

When patients in whom ventricular arrhythmias increased during daily activities underwent stress testing, slight exercising without load or with loads below 300 kg precipitated frequent runs of uniform or multiform ventricular tachycardia (VT) (Fig. 8-3 *B*). Thus, arrhythmogenic mechanisms are clearly enhanced by even a slight increase in adrenergic tone. To rule out the possibility that these changes in ventricular ectopic activity are simply related to changes in heart rate, we compared the effect of the increase of heart rate during sinus rhythm (due to exercise) with similar or equal rates obtained by atrial pacing. After recovery from exercise, atrial pacing at a similar cycle length did not trigger ventricular ectopic activity (Fig. 8-3 *C*).

Only rarely have we observed increments of ventricular ectopic activity during sleep or at rest. This may indicate that the arrhythmogenic mechanisms are associated with slower heart rates, which probably favor dispersion of ventricular refractoriness, or with rate-dependent conduction disturbances (bradycardia-dependent block). In conclusion, a significant number of patients are supersensitive to changes in autonomic tone, whereas others are partially or totally unaffected. Thus, the propensity for development of dangerous ventricular arrhythmias and sudden cardiac death is closely related to this phenomenon.

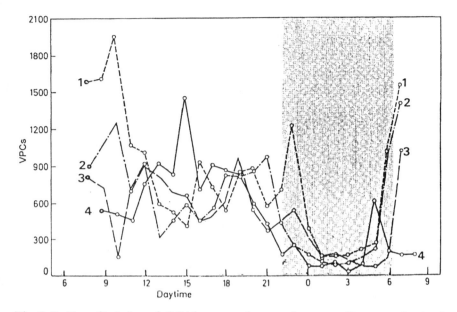

Fig. 8-2. Four (1, 2, 3, and 4) 24-hour continuous electrocardiograms obtained at weekly intervals in a patient with chronic chagasic cardiomyopathy. Reproducibility of the hourly distribution shows strikingly similar behavior during the 24 hours (except for brief periods). The four Holter recordings show a similarly marked circadian variation. The shaded area represents the sleeping hours. The ordinate indicates the number of ventricular premature contractions (VPCs), and the abscissa shows the hour distribution during 24-hour ambulatory Holter recording.

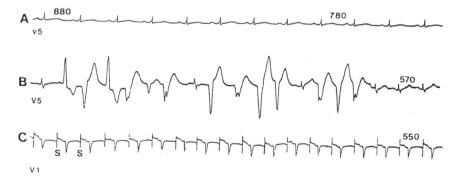

Fig. 8-3. Exercise-related complex ventricular arrhythmias in a chagasic patient. *A*, Rhythm strip obtained at rest. No ventricular premature contractions are present with RR intervals during sinus rhythm between 780 and 880 msec. *B*, During slight exercise, chaotic ventricular activity develops when the RR intervals shorten to 570 msec. *C*, Transesophageal atrial pacing (S) at equal or even shorter RR intervals does not trigger ventricular ectopic beats.

Spontaneous Variability of Potentially Malignant Ventricular Arrhythmias

A group of patients had potentially malignant ventricular arrhythmias that were strikingly persistent and steady.[21] Short-, intermediate-, and long-term variabilities were assessed. In an investigation of short-term variability during a 24-hour period, 8 of 16 patients without significant circadian variations had a maximal hourly reduction in the number of VPCs (compared with the number in the first hour of recording) of less than 50%. Conversely, in 8 of 12 patients with sharp circadian variations, the maximal hourly reduction in the number of VPCs at rest was greater than 90%. If resting hours were excluded in the latter group of patients, the degree of spontaneous variation was similar to that in the former group. A close correlation was observed between the number of VPCs and the occurrence of couplets, nonsustained VT, and R on T phenomenon. However, as previously stated, multiformity was a constant finding in all patients, even those with the fewest VPCs.

For exploration of intermediate-term and long-term spontaneous variability, 24-hour ambulatory Holter recordings were obtained at weekly intervals during 4 weeks and at 10 and 24 months after the first study (Fig. 8-2). The maximum changes ranged between +39% and –39% in the intermediate-term studies and +57.6% and –59.1% in the long-term evaluations. As in the short-term studies, the spontaneous variability of couplets, runs of VT, and R on T phenomenon paralleled those described for the total number of VPCs. These observations are in contrast to data from studies in patients with frequent VPCs caused by other cardiomyopathies or ischemic heart disease,[27-29] in whom spontaneous variability is much greater than in patients with CChM.

We found that because of this remarkable persistence and stability of ventricular arrhythmias, they allow an accurate evaluation of antiarrhythmic treatments and largely exclude the therapeutic or proarrhythmic effects mimicked by spontaneous variability.[27] Consequently, the ventricular arrhythmias of patients with CChM constitute a reliable model to test the efficacy of antiarrhythmic drugs in these arrhythmias and to evaluate their potential usefulness for prevention of sudden cardiac death. However, this "chagasic model" is particularly demanding, because in patients with the severe underlying myocardial damage that serves as the anatomical substrate for these arrhythmias, many antiarrhythmic drugs may be both ineffective and dangerous (because of deleterious hemodynamic and electrophysiologic effects). We may confidently predict that any drug passing this difficult test can be used in any other cardiac condition leading to these or other arrhythmias.

Electrophysiologic Mechanisms of Ventricular Arrhythmias

CChM includes a wide variety of anatomical and electrophysiologic alterations that lead to the many kinds of atrial and ventricular arrhythmias. Widespread fibrosis may disrupt cell contacts, impairing propagation of impulses.[30] Cardiac dilatation and hypertrophy may also affect connections between cells (and favor subendocardial ischemia).[31] Moreover, myocardial ischemia and microvascular dysfunction[9,10] have been postulated to be implicated in the pathogenesis of the myocardial lesions of CChM. They may induce shifting of the resting potential to less negative values, prolongation of the duration of the action potential, and disruption of cell contacts.[32] In addition, hypertrophy and dilatation may induce early afterdepolarizations and other abnormalities in impulse formation.[33] Altogether, these anatomical and electrophysiologic alterations may produce inhomogeneities in repolarization and refractoriness in various areas of the ventricles, resulting in slowing of conduction, unidirectional block, and reentry.

Pharmacologic Treatment

Class I Drugs

In the early 1960s, we knew that ventricular arrhythmias in CChM were dangerous and that they were related to sudden cardiac death. Since at that time only quinidine and procainamide were available, we used these drugs to treat some very symptomatic patients with complex ventricular arrhythmias. Soon after, we learned that these arrhythmias worsened, and two patients died suddenly during the administration of the drug. Our conclusion was that quinidine or any other drug with similar electrophysiologic properties might be proarrhythmic in patients with severe structural heart disease like that in advanced forms of CChM. Since then, we have totally avoided the use of quinidine and quinidine-like drugs for the treatment of chagasic ventricular arrhythmias in our center.

At present, it is well known that class I agents may be associated with an increased risk of proarrhythmia in patients with structural heart disease, such as that occurring in the Cardiac Arrhythmia Suppression Trial[34] despite a striking suppression of ventricular ectopy. Class I drugs block sodium channels and decrease the rate of increase of phase 0 of the action potential, further slowing conduction velocity and predisposing to reentry. On the other hand, quinidine and quinidine-like drugs may induce early afterdepolarizations and torsades de pointes. The latter effect may be even more prominent in the M cells located in the midmyocardial layers.[33]

In conclusion, quinidine, procainamide, and class IC agents (flecainide, encainide, moricizine, and propafenone) may generate arrhythmogenesis in CChM. As in any other cardiac disease, a low ejection fraction (40% or less) may also increase the risk of proarrhythmia.

Class II Drugs

Class II antiarrhythmic drugs have not been systematically studied in patients with CChM and ventricular arrhythmias. The high incidences of sick sinus syndrome, atrioventricular node compromise, and cardiac failure among patients with CChM have been the main limitations for their use; hence, there are no reports of their effects on survival or antiarrhythmic action. Patients with potentially malignant ventricular arrhythmias clearly related to an increased adrenergic drive of the heart and without cardiac failure may benefit from oral administration of β-adrenergic blockers. As a test of this assumption, 10 patients with adrenergic-related complex ventricular arrhythmias and normal or near-normal left ventricular function were sequentially treated with propranolol, d,l-sotalol, and amiodarone (unpublished personal observations). All patients had 24-hour continuous recordings before, during, and after receiving each drug. Surprisingly, propranolol did not have any significant effect on the number and complexity of ventricular arrhythmias (couplets, nonsustained VT, and R on T phenomenon).

d,l-Sotalol (which is actually a class III antiarrhythmic drug with β-blocking properties) caused a significant reduction in VPCs (80.2%) and almost total suppression of couplets and nonsustained VT. Amiodarone almost totally suppressed ventricular ectopy (97.58%) and completely abolished couplets and VT in all patients. The mild effect of propranolol cannot be extrapolated to all β-blockers. In fact, many years ago we assessed the antiarrhythmic action of nadolol in five patients with CChM in whom ventricular arrhythmias were worsened by sympathetic discharge.[35] In three of the five patients, nadolol abolished ventricular arrhythmias, which could no longer be elicited during repeated stress tests in a follow-up period of 2 to 6 months. Thus, in our experience, nadolol and d,l-sotalol might be considered useful alternative therapeutic agents. Further studies are necessary in a larger number of patients to determine the efficacy and safety of β-adrenergic blocking agents in chagasic ventricular arrhythmias.

Comparative Effects of Classes I, III, and IV Drugs

To further test the antiarrhythmic action of different classes of agents, we used serial 24-hour ambulatory Holter recordings to evaluate comparatively the effects of four antiarrhythmic drugs with different electrophysiologic properties—mexiletine, 17-monochloroacetylajmaline, amiodarone, and verapamil—in 14 chagasic patients with severe and persistent ventricular arrhythmias.[36] According to the study protocol, drugs and their placebos were administered orally in the following order: placebo and verapamil, placebo and mexiletine, placebo and 17-monochloroacetylajmaline (1 week each), and, finally, placebo and amiodarone (4 weeks each). A 24-hour ambulatory Holter recording was obtained after administration of each placebo and drug. Although plasma concentrations were not measured, the doses used were known to produce effective levels in the treatment of other arrhythmias and the period of administration of the drugs was greater than five half-lives (except for amiodarone). Of note, side effects occurred only during drug treatment and not during placebo administration.

On the basis of the results of this study, the pharmacologic responses to these drugs are analyzed separately.

Antiarrhythmic Response to Verapamil

All patients received a daily dose of 320 mg of verapamil during a week. Treatment with verapamil was associated with nonsignificant reductions in the total number of VPCs (30.8%), couplets (18.6%), and runs of ventricular tachycardia (30.9%). Likewise, multiform VPCs and the R on T phenomenon remained unmodified without significant changes. Total suppression of nonsustained VT was achieved in only 1 of 11 patients (9.09%), and couplets and VPCs persisted in all 14 patients (Fig. 8-4). The most serious side effect of verapamil was congestive heart failure, which occurred in three patients. Obviously, this complication was interpreted as a detrimental effect of the drug on cardiac contractile performance. Marked sinus bradycardia or sinoatrial block developed in 11 of the 14 patients, either at rest or during the sleeping hours (fewer than 40 beats per minute). The high incidence of severe sinus depression induced by verapamil was indirect evidence of a latent dysfunction of this structure, which has been reported as frequent.[37,38]

Verapamil exerts its effects by blocking the L-type calcium channels. Its failure to control the ventricular arrhythmias of CChM or

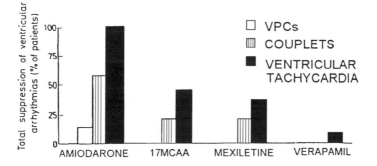

Fig. 8-4. Percentage of patients with total suppression of ventricular arrhythmias during treatment with amiodarone, 7-monochloroacetylajmaline (17MCAA), mexiletine, and verapamil (see text). VPCs, ventricular premature contractions.

to induce or aggravate intraventricular conduction disturbances (at baseline, 12 of the 14 patients had intraventricular conduction defects) suggests that slow responses do not have a significant function, if any, in the mechanisms of chagasic ventricular arrhythmias and conduction disturbances.

Response to Sodium Channel Blocking Agents

In the same study,[36] mexiletine and 17-monochloroacetylajmaline were administered at daily doses of 800 mg and 1,200 mg, respectively, during 1 week each. Both drugs were similarly noneffective in reducing the number of VPCs but significantly reduced runs of VT and couplets. With mexiletine, runs of VT and couplets were suppressed in 86.4% and 87.7%, respectively, and with 17-monochloroacetylajmaline, these arrhythmias were reduced in 78.3% and 73.6%. Thus, complex forms and VT were totally suppressed in a small, nonsignificant percentage of cases (Fig. 8-4), and multiform VPCs remained constant. The R on T phenomenon was suppressed in 42.8% and 28.5% of patients during administration of mexiletine and 17-monochloroacetylajmaline, respectively.

Mexiletine induced marked sinus bradycardia and transient sino-atrial block in 7 patients, and 17-monochloroacetylajmaline had the same effects in 10 patients. In addition, transient right bundle branch block was induced by mexiletine in four patients and during 17-mono-chloroacetylajmaline treatment in three of these four patients.

The moderate antiarrhythmic effect and the induction of intraventricular conduction defects by these drugs indicate that both ventricular arrhythmias and conduction disturbances in patients with CChM are probably related to depressed fast responses. The relatively weak antiarrhythmic effect may be related to a rather feeble blockade of the sodium channel. However, more powerful blockers of the sodium channels, flecainide and propafenone, were found to have antiarrhythmic action similar to that of mexiletine and 17-monochloroacetylajmaline (unpublished personal observations).

Efficacy of Amiodarone

In a study by Haedo et al.,[36] amiodarone, a unique wide-spectrum antiarrhythmic agent, controlled the ventricular arrhythmias better than did sodium and calcium channel blockers. After 4 weeks of amiodarone administration at a daily dose of 800 mg, isolated VPCs and complex forms of VPCs were significantly suppressed. The average reduction of VPCs was 97.8%, and two patients had total suppression of ventricular ectopy. VT was abolished in all patients. Couplets were reduced by 98.1%, with complete suppression in half the patients (57.14%) (Fig. 8-4). The R on T phenomenon was abolished in 78.5%

of the patients. However, the multiform pattern of VPCs was not significantly affected. Amiodarone also induced bradycardia and sinoatrial block in eight patients and, like mexiletine and 17-monochloroacetylajmaline, induced transient right bundle branch block in three patients.

Amiodarone was the most effective of the four tested drugs. The mechanisms causing its powerful antiarrhythmic action remain only partially understood. Amiodarone is a singular agent, with classes I, II, III, and IV effects. Probably the most striking electrophysiologic property of amiodarone is the ability to prolong the duration of action potentials in ventricular fibers of the endocardium and epicardium, with lesser effects in Purkinje cells[39] and M cells,[40] thus reducing transmural dispersion of refractoriness. Moreover, amiodarone has been shown to be capable of eliminating the tendency for the development of early afterdepolarization in Purkinje and M cells.[41,42] In addition, another distinctive electrophysiologic property could help abolish ventricular arrhythmias. It has been shown that amiodarone causes a significant lengthening of the absolute refractory period at the expense of the relative refractory period of the normal Purkinje and muscular fibers.[43] Thus, premature stimulation would produce either total block or normal propagation, suppressing slow conduction necessary for reentrant or reflecting mechanisms. Amiodarone is also an effective anti-ischemic drug, with an excellent hemodynamic profile[44-49] and a low incidence of ventricular proarrhythmia. In fact, it is well known that despite slowing the heart rate and prolonging the QTc interval, amiodarone has the lowest propensity for reproducing torsades de pointes.[50] In our comparative study, amiodarone was the only drug causing a significant and consistent slowing of the mean sinus node rate, an effect that may also account for an additional factor contributing to its greater antiarrhythmic action. However, even in patients without significant bradycardiac effect, amiodarone strongly reduced ventricular ectopy, even when heart rates were relatively fast.[26]

Long-Term Evaluation of Antiarrhythmic Efficacy

The comparative antiarrhythmic efficacy of amiodarone in the study by Haedo et al.[36] occurred during short-term administration. However, the treatment of chagasic ventricular arrhythmias must be long-lasting, and long-term evaluation is thus required to confidently evaluate the efficacy and safety of the drug and its clinical implications for symptoms and fatal arrhythmic events.

Chiale et al.[51] studied the results of long-term administration of amiodarone in 24 patients with CChM and severe ventricular arrhythmias. Eight of the 24 patients had experienced syncope, and 2 others complained of dizziness. Seven patients had cardiac failure. Serial 24-hour ambulatory Holter recordings were obtained in all patients at the control stage, and amiodarone was given orally at daily doses of 600 to 800 mg. Holter recordings were repeated at weekly intervals, and the dose was increased (if necessary) to 800 to 1,000 mg/day if repetitive forms (couplets or VT) were not totally eliminated. When the maximal antiarrhythmic effect was attained (mean, 7.4 ± 1 weeks) (Fig. 8-5), continuous 24-hour recordings were spaced out to intervals of every 15 to 90 days until completion of 6 months of treatment. Afterward, the recordings were obtained every 3 to 6 months. The mean follow-up period was 26.6 months.

The frequency of VPCs in the control studies was between 3,780 and 61,733 in 24 hours (mean, 17,137 ± 3,055). All patients had multiform ventricular ectopic beats and countless couplets. Nonsustained VT was present in 21 patients. The VT was uniform in 5 patients and multiform in 16. The R on T phenomenon was observed in 17 patients. In 14 patients, the frequency of VPCs was persistently high all day, whereas 9 patients had a substantial reduction during the sleeping hours.

In 23 of the 24 patients, substantial and sustained reduction (93.2% to 99.9%; mean, 94.8%) in the number of VPCs was documented (Fig. 8-5 and 8-6). Of note, ventricular couplets were totally eliminated in 22 of 24 patients (92%), and the runs of VT were suppressed in 20 of 21 (95%). The R on T phenomenon was abolished in 15 of 17 patients (88%), and multiformity of ventricular extrasystoles was not significantly reduced. Only two patients had no response to amiodarone treatment (indicated by stars in Fig. 8-6). In one, couplets and salvos of VT persisted despite a clear reduction in the number of VPCs (98%). This patient died suddenly during amiodarone treatment. The other

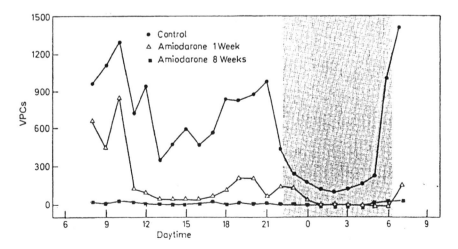

Fig. 8-5. The maximal antiarrhythmic effect of amiodarone is obtained after 8 weeks of treatment. In the ordinate, the numbers indicate the number of ventricular premature contractions (VPCs). In the abscissa, the hour distribution during 24-hour ambulatory Holter recording is shown. The shaded area indicates the sleeping hours.

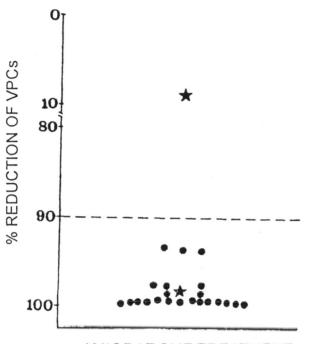

AMIODARONE TREATMENT

Fig. 8-6. Long-term antiarrhythmic effect of amiodarone in 24 patients with chronic chagasic cardiomyopathy and potentially malignant ventricular arrhythmias. Reduction of more than 80% in the number of ventricular premature contractions (VPCs) occurred in 23 patients (*dots*). The *stars* represent two patients without a response in whom repetitive VPCs persisted.

patient did not have any significant response to the antiarrhythmic therapy.

During follow-up, four patients died. One died of recurrent pulmonary embolism. One experienced sudden death during the fifth month of treatment, the day after a Holter recording showed 125 VPCs, several couplets, and one symptomatic episode of nonsustained VT (17 seconds). The third patient died during acute pulmonary edema, and the fourth committed suicide. In seven of the eight patients with syncope, the crises were completely eliminated. None of the seven patients with cardiac failure experienced aggravation of the hemodynamic condition.

Dose-Response Relationship

Ventricular arrhythmias were controlled in 9 of the 24 patients with the initial dose of 600 to 800 mg. In some patients, the dose had to be increased to 800 to 1,000 mg/day to achieve satisfactory control of ventricular arrhythmias. Altogether, the mean dose to attain the maximal antiarrhythmic effect was 782 mg/day. The maximal antiarrhythmic effect of the drug was defined as the one occurring whenever two or more consecutive 24-hour ambulatory ECG recordings showed a mean intervariation in the number of VPCs, couplets, and VT episodes of less than 2.5%. In four patients, the dose of amiodarone was lowered to 600 or 400 mg/day when the expected antiarrhythmic action was attained.[51]

Because of the well-known cumulative action of amiodarone, the maximal antiarrhythmic effect was achieved gradually, after 3 to 26 weeks (mean, 7.4 weeks), and discontinuance after several months of uninterrupted administration of amiodarone showed that its suppressing effect on repetitive forms of the ventricular arrhythmia persisted 28 to 45 days. If the response of chagasic ventricular arrhythmias to amiodarone is compared with the responses of other clinical arrhythmias (atrial tachyarrhythmias, ventricular arrhythmias related to ischemic heart disease, and idiopathic cardiomyopathies), it is apparent that the chagasic are the least sensitive.[52] On the other hand, this is an indirect way of emphasizing the severity of the ventricular arrhythmias in CChM.

Control of Potentially Malignant Ventricular Arrhythmias and Sudden Death

To date, there are no properly programmed prospective trials in larger groups of chagasic patients to ascertain whether pharmacologic control of potentially ventricular arrhythmias helps prevent sudden cardiac death. In accordance with Rosenbaum's opinion,[3] it has been estimated that about 20% of patients with advanced forms of CChM die within 2 years after the diagnosis has been made. In the report by Chiale et al.,[51] the rate of mortality imputable to CChM in the 22 patients with a response to amiodarone was significantly lower (9%) during the mean 26.6-month follow-up.

Cardiac Side Effects

Two of the 24 patients receiving the drug had marked sinus bradycardia during sleep; one had occasional episodes of sinoatrial block, and two had right bundle branch block. In one patient whose disease evolved to symptomatic second-degree atrioventricular block after 3 years of treatment, the event was interpreted as a simple manifestation of the natural course of the disease. As previously stated, none of the patients appeared to have aggravation of ventricular function. On the contrary, probably because ventricular arrhythmias were controlled and the cardiac rate was slowed, a significant hemodynamic improvement was observed in three patients with overt heart failure at the time of inclusion.[51]

Noncardiac Side Effects

In one patient, thyrotoxicosis developed simultaneously with exacerbation of arrhythmia after 10 months of treatment. Thyroid dysfunction was successfully controlled, and administration of amiodarone was not discontinued. Facial discoloration was observed in two patients, and corneal microdeposits were detected in all patients without worsening of visual acuity. Gastric discomfort and constipation were referred to by a nonsignificant number of patients. Despite the side effects mentioned here, none of these patients discontinued treatment.[51] Special attention was paid to the detection of interstitial pneumonitis, which rarely occurs.[53,54]

Combined Pharmacologic Therapy

Although amiodarone has been shown to be the most powerful and safest antiarrhythmic drug, control of ventricular arrhythmias cannot be satisfactorily achieved in some patients with CChM. Thus, because of either true refractoriness of the arrhythmia or unbearable side effects that preclude the use of high doses of the drug, a combination of two antiarrhythmic drugs may be warranted to obtain greater antiarrhythmic activity or to reduce or eliminate side effects. However, some combinations of antiarrhythmic drugs in chagasic patients, such as the association of amiodarone with β-blockers, can easily induce serious cardiac side effects, including deterioration of the hemodynamic conditions.

So far, we have tried two associations. One is combining low doses of amiodarone (200 to 300 mg/day) and mexiletine (600 to 720 mg/day) in previously treated patients who had a poor antiarrhythmic response or intolerable secondary effects. This combined treatment has been particularly useful in controlling ventricular arrhythmias and improving tolerance (unpublished observations).

Another association frequently used in our center is the simultaneous administration of d,l-sotalol and mexiletine. Unpublished observations (in 10 chagasic patients with malignant ventricular arrhythmias) have clearly shown that the antiarrhythmic effect of d,l-sotalol is highly potentiated after the addition of oral mexiletine. Moreover, in vivo[55] and in vitro[56] experimental studies showed that mexiletine may exert an additional benefit when used with d,l-sotalol by controlling inappropriate prolongation of the action potential of M cells, which may give rise to early afterdepolarizations.[56]

Nonconventional Medical Treatment of Ventricular Arrhythmias

In recent years, it has been proposed that ventricular arrhythmias and bradyarrhythmias in CChM and idiopathic dilated cardiomyopathy may be related to antibodies with agonist-like properties on the autonomic β-adrenergic and M_2-cholinergic membrane receptors of cardiac cells, respectively.[8,57-59]

Enhanced sympathetic drive of the heart might be important in the pathophysiology of ventricular tachyarrhythmias,[60,61] and, conversely, augmented vagal tone may depress sinus node activity as well as atrioventricular nodal conduction.[62,63] Since both types of antibodies are highly prevalent in patients with CChM who have ventricular arrhythmias and sinus node dysfunction, it may be postulated that these arrhythmias might be prevented or controlled by immunoadsorption, a procedure that eliminates the antibodies from circulation for relatively long periods.[64] In fact, Müller et al.[65] observed that the most severe ventricular arrhythmias in patients with idiopathic dilated cardiomyopathy and circulating anti-$β_1$-adrenergic receptor antibodies could be prevented by immunoadsorption. Although this procedure has not yet been tried in chagasic patients, we may well assume that similar results could be obtained.

Atrial Arrhythmias

As stated, the sinus node and the atria are commonly involved in CChM, and the result may be atrial extrasystoles, severe depression of sinus node activity, sinoatrial block, bradycardia-tachycardia syndrome, and atrial fibrillation or flutter.

The prevalence of sinus node dysfunction in infected persons depends on the period of infection and the clinical form of CChM. Sinus node dysfunction and atrial arrhythmias have not been reported during the acute period, except for atrial extrasystoles and atrial tachycardia in the rare instances of severe acute myocarditis.[2,3]

In CChM, most patients with sick sinus syndrome also have atrioventricular node involvement (binodal disease).[15] In manifest CChM, the prevalence of sinus node dysfunction is high, and the most frequent manifestation is persistent and usually severe sinus bradycardia, even in heart failure. Sinus arrest or sinoatrial block is commonly observed under these circumstances. Frequently, atropine or isoproterenol infusion and exercise show that these patients cannot increase heart rate.[15]

Prolonged cardiac asystole is uncommon because of enhanced atrial or ventricular subsidiary pacemaker activity, probably from cellular injury, and overdrive excitation of subsidiary atrial pacemakers is not unusual.[15] Although isolated atrial extrasystoles occur, atrial tachycardias are, in our experience, strikingly uncommon. Despite the high prevalence of sinus node dysfunction in CChM, the typical bradycardia-tachycardia syndrome is not as frequent as one would expect. The low incidence of this syndrome is probably related to the autonomic denervation of the heart, which commonly occurs in chronic Chagas' heart disease.[11,12] Since cholinergic and adrenergic stimuli are thought to precipitate most of these arrhythmias, it is feasible to postulate that "cardiac denervation" in chagasic patients may, to some extent, prevent the arrhythmogenic action of the autonomic nervous system reflexes.

In CChM, the association of sinus bradycardia and sinus node dysfunction with potentially malignant ventricular arrhythmias is strikingly common. This combination precludes the use of antiarrhythmic drugs that may aggravate sinus bradycardia unless a permanent pacemaker is implanted. In the advanced stages of the disease with marked dilatation of both ventricles and enlargement of the left atrium, permanent atrial fibrillation or flutter is often observed.

Atrial tachyarrhythmias are exceptional in CChM without moderate to severe ventricular damage, but in the advanced stages of the disease, ventricular arrhythmias are almost invariably present. Thus, as in our preceding consideration of the pharmacologic therapy of ventricular arrhythmias, amiodarone is the first choice and safest drug for the treatment or prevention of atrial arrhythmias when they deserve to be treated. However, sinus node dysfunction, atrioventricular nodal delay, and intraventricular conduction delay frequently contraindicate the use of this agent unless a permanent pacemaker is implanted.

Class II drugs have also very limited use for the treatment of atrial arrhythmias in CChM because of the high prevalence of sinus bradycardia and cardiac failure. In turn, class I agents (particularly class IC) may be proarrhythmic because of the anatomical and electrophysiologic substrate of the arrhythmias in Chagas' heart disease. It is now well known that the slowing of conduction induced by these drugs predisposes to the possibility of reentry and proarrhythmia in a structurally abnormal heart.[34]

Clinical Implications

An estimated 16 to 18 million people are infected with *Trypanosoma cruzi*, and 90 million are at risk of infection. In turn, about 20% of infected persons have CChM, and many of them are at risk of sudden death. The availability of antiarrhythmic drugs capable of preventing, at least in part, this complication is of the utmost importance. The results of different studies disclosed in this chapter suggest that amiodarone alone or in combination with mexiletine, and probably also *d,l*-sotalol combined with mexiletine, may be extremely effective against the most dangerous ventricular arrhythmias of CChM and may eventually prevent the occurrence of sudden arrhythmic death, as shown for cardiac diseases of other causes.[48,66-68]

The implantable cardioverter-defibrillator has been used in many chagasic patients with sustained monomorphic VT and hemodynamic compromise or after resuscitation from ventricular fibrillation. Because most of these patients have concomitant severe left or global ventricular dysfunction, indications for this device are often seriously limited. Although use of the implantable cardioverter-defibrillator has not been compared with a pharmacologic approach in a randomized study in chagasic patients with life-threatening arrhythmias, it is conceivable that this device either alone or in combination with an effective antiarrhythmic agent would benefit many of these patients by suppressing most of the arrhythmias without fear of death from proarrhythmia.[69]

Chagas' disease is related to strong cultural, social, and economic conditions. Hence, the most advanced and expensive medical resources are not always feasible for a high percentage of the approximately 45,000 persons who die each year because of CChM, the most frequent specific cardiomyopathy.[70]

References

1. Pan American Health Organization: Health Conditions in the Americas, 1990 Edition, Scientific publication 524, Vol 1. Washington, DC, Pan American Health Organization, Pan American Sanitary Bureau, Regional Office of the World Health Organization, 1990, pp 160-164
2. Laranja FS, Dias E, Nobrega G, Miranda A: Chagas' disease; a clinical, epidemiologic, and pathologic study. Circulation 14:1035-1060, 1956
3. Rosenbaum MB: Chagasic cardiomyopathy. Prog Cardiovasc Dis 7:199-225, 1964
4. Amorim DS: Chagas' disease. In Progress in Cardiology. Vol 8. Edited by PN Yu, JF Goodwin. Philadelphia, Lea & Febiger, 1979, pp 235-279
5. Sachs RN, Lanfranchi J: Primary cardiomyopathies and immunologic disorders [French]. Coeur Med Interne 17:193-198, 1978
6. Ribeiro Dos Santos R, Hudson L: Trypanosoma cruzi: immunological consequences of parasite modification of host cells. Clin Exp Immunol 40:36-41, 1980
7. Peralta JM, Ginefra P, Dias JC, Magalhaes JM, Szarfman A: Autoantibodies and chronic Chagas's heart disease. Trans R Soc Trop Med Hyg 75:568-569, 1981
8. Rosenbaum MB, Chiale PA, Schejtman D, Levin M, Elizari MV: Antibodies to beta-adrenergic receptors disclosing agonist-like properties in idiopathic dilated cardiomyopathy and Chagas' heart disease. J Cardiovasc Electrophysiol 5:367-375, 1994
9. Morris SA, Tanowitz HB, Wittner M, Bilezikian JP: Pathophysiological insights into the cardiomyopathy of Chagas' disease. Circulation 82:1900-1909, 1990
10. Torres FW, Acquatella H, Condado J, Dinsmore R, Palacios IF: Endothelium dependent coronary vasomotion is abnormal in patients with Chagas heart disease (abstract). J Am Coll Cardiol 21 Suppl:197A, 1993
11. Mott KE, Hagstrom JW: The pathologic lesions of the cardiac autonomic nervous system in chronic Chagas' myocarditis. Circulation 31:273-286, 1965
12. Oliveira JS: A natural human model of intrinsic heart nervous system denervation: Chagas' cardiopathy. Am Heart J 110:1092-1098, 1985
13. Mengel JO, Rossi MA: Chronic chagasic myocarditis pathogenesis: dependence on autoimmune and microvascular factors. Am Heart J 124:1052-1057, 1992

14. Oliveira JS, Mello De Oliveira JA, Frederigue U Jr, Lima Filho EC: Apical aneurysm of Chagas's heart disease. Br Heart J 46:432-437, 1981
15. Elizari MV, Chiale PA: Cardiac arrhythmias in Chagas' heart disease. J Cardiovasc Electrophysiol 4:596-608, 1993
16. Prata A: Natural history of chagasic cardiomyopathy. In American Trypanosomiasis Research. Washington, DC, Pan American Health Organization, 1975, p 191
17. Reis Lopes E, Chapadeiro E, Almeida HC, Rocha A: Contribucao ao estudo de anatomia patologica dos coracoes de chagásicos falecidos subitamente. Rev Soc Bras Med Trop 9:269-279, 1976
18. de Paola AA, Horowitz LN, Miyamoto MH, Pinheiro R, Ferreira DF, Terzian AB, Cirenza C, Guiguer N Jr, Portugal OP: Angiographic and electrophysiologic substrates of ventricular tachycardia in chronic Chagasic myocarditis. Am J Cardiol 65:360-363, 1990
19. Carrasco Guerra HA: Prognostic value of complex arrhythmias in chagasic patients. X World Cardiology Congress, Washington, 1986, Abstract 676
20. Bigger JT Jr: Definition of benign versus malignant ventricular arrhythmias: targets for treatment. Am J Cardiol 52:47C-54C, 1983
21. Chiale PA, Halpern MS, Nau GJ, Przybylski J, Tambussi AM, Lazzari JO, Elizari MV, Rosenbaum MB: Malignant ventricular arrhythmias in chronic chagasic myocarditis. Pacing Clin Electrophysiol 5:162-172, 1982
22. Kaski JC, Girotti LA, Messuti H, Rutitzky B, Rosenbaum MB: Long-term management of sustained, recurrent, symptomatic ventricular tachycardia with amiodarone. Circulation 64:273-279, 1981
23. Case records of the Massachusetts General Hospital (Case 32-1993). N Engl J Med 329:488-496, 1993
24. Hagar JM, Rahimtoola SH: Chagas' heart disease in the United States. N Engl J Med 325:763-768, 1991
25. Maguire JH, Hoff R, Sherlock I, Guimaraes AC, Sleigh AC, Ramos NB, Mott KE, Weller TH: Cardiac morbidity and mortality due to Chagas' disease: Prospective electrocardiographic study of a Brazilian community. Circulation 75:1140-1145, 1987
26. Chiale PA, Rosenbaum MB: Clinical and pharmacologic characterization and treatment of potentially malignant arrhythmias of chronic chagasic cardiomyopathy. In Handbook of Experimental Pharmacology: Antiarrhythmic Drugs, Vol 89. Edited by EM Vaughan Williams, TJ Campbell. Berlin, Springer-Verlag, 1989, pp 601-620
27. Winkle RA: Antiarrhythmic drug effect mimicked by spontaneous variability of ventricular ectopy. Circulation 57:1116-1121, 1978
28. Winkle RA, Meffin PJ, Harrison DC: Long-term tocainide therapy for ventricular arrhythmias. Circulation 57:1008-1016, 1978
29. Winkle RA, Gradman AH, Fitzgerald JW: Antiarrhythmic drug effect assessed from ventricular arrhythmia reduction in the ambulatory electrocardiogram and treadmill test: comparison of propranolol, procainamide and quinidine. Am J Cardiol 42:473-480, 1978
30. Spach MS, Boineau JP: Microfibrosis produces electrical load variations due to loss of side-to-side cell connections: a major mechanism of structural heart disease arrhythmias. Pacing Clin Electrophysiol 20:397-413, 1997
31. Goodwin JF: Congestive and hypertrophic cardiomyopathies. A decade of study. Lancet 1:731-739, 1970

32. Pogwizd SM, Corr PB: Reentrant and nonreentrant mechanisms contribute to arrhythmogenesis during early myocardial ischemia: results using three-dimensional mapping. Circ Res 61:352-371, 1987

33. Antzelevitch C, Sicouri S: Clinical relevance of cardiac arrhythmias generated by after depolarizations. Role of M cells in the generation of U waves, triggered activity and torsade de pointes. J Am Coll Cardiol 23:259-277, 1994

34. The Cardiac Arrhythmia Suppression Trial (CAST) Investigators: Preliminary report: effect of encainide and flecainide on mortality in a randomized trial of arrhythmia suppression after myocardial infarction. N Engl J Med 321:406-412, 1989

35. Schmidberg JM, Acunzo RM, Nau GJ, Elizari MV, Rosenbaum MB: Eficacia del nadalol en el tratamiento de las arritmias ventriculares inducidas o agravadas por la ergometría (abstract). Rev Arg Cardiol 53:S130, 1985

36. Haedo AH, Chiale PA, Bandieri JD, Lazzari JO, Elizari MV, Rosenbaum MB: Comparative antiarrhythmic efficacy of verapamil, 17-monochloracetylajmaline, mexiletine and amiodarone in patients with severe chagasic myocarditis: relation with the underlying arrhythmogenic mechanisms. J Am Coll Cardiol 7:1114-1120, 1986

37. Andrade ZA, Camara EJ, Sadigursky M, Andrade SG: Sinus node involvement in Chagas' disease [Portuguese]. Arq Bras Cardiol 50:153-158, 1988

38. Carrasco HA, Mora R, Inglessis G, Contreras JM, Marval J, Fuenmayor A: Study of sinus node function and atrioventricular conduction in patients with Chagas disease [Spanish]. Arch Inst Cardiol Mex 52:245-251, 1982

39. Papp JG, Nemeth M, Krassoi I, et al: Differential electrophysiologic effects of chronically administered amiodarone on canine Purkinje fibers versus ventricular muscle. J Pharmacol Exp Ther 1:187-196, 1996

40. Sicouri S, Moro S, Litovsky S, Elizari MV, Antzelevitch C: Chronic amiodarone reduces transmural dispersion of repolarization in the canine heart. J Cardiovasc Electrophysiol 8:1269-1279, 1997

41. Kodama I, Kamiya K, Toyama J: Cellular electropharmacology of amiodarone. Cardiovasc Res 35:13-29, 1997

42. Sicouri S, Moro S, Elizari MV: d-Sotalol induces marked action potential prolongation and early afterdepolarizations in M but not epicardial or endocardial cells of the canine ventricle. J Cardiovasc Pharmacol Therapeut 2:27-38, 1997

43. Elizari MV, Levi RJ, Novakosky A, Lazzari JO, Vetulli HM: Cellular effects of antiarrhythmic drugs. Remarks on methodology. In Symposium on Antiarrhythmic and Antianginal Drugs with Cumulative Effects. Paris, SANOFI Pharmaceutical, 1980, pp 9-23

44. Cleland JG, Dargie HJ, Ford I: Mortality in heart failure: clinical variables of prognostic value. Br Heart J 58:572-582, 1987

45. Nicklas JM, McKenna WJ, Stewart RA, Mickelson JK, Das SK, Schork MA, Krikler SJ, Quain LA, Morady F, Pitt B: Prospective, double-blind, placebo-controlled trial of low-dose amiodarone in patients with severe heart failure and asymptomatic frequent ventricular ectopy. Am Heart J 122:1016-1021, 1991

46. Stevenson WG, Stevenson LW, Middlekauff HR, Fonarow GC, Hamilton MA, Woo MA, Saxon LA, Natterson PD, Steimle A, Walden JA, Tillisch JH: Improving survival for patients with atrial fibrillation and advanced heart failure. J Am Coll Cardiol 28:1458-1463, 1996

47. Hamer AW, Arkles LB, Johns JA: Beneficial effects of low dose amiodarone in patients with congestive cardiac failure: a placebo-controlled trial. J Am Coll Cardiol 14:1768-1774, 1989

48. Doval HC, Nul DR, Grancelli HO, Perrone SV, Bortman GR, Curiel R for Grupo de Estudio de la Sobrevida en la Insuficiencia Cardiaca en Argentina: Randomized trial of low-dose amiodarone in severe congestive heart failure. Lancet 344:493-498, 1994

49. Singh SN, Fletcher RD, Fisher SG, Singh BN, Lewis HD, Deedwania PC, Massie BM, Colling C, Lazzeri D, for the Survival Trial of Antiarrhythmic Therapy in Congestive Heart Failure: Amiodarone in patients with congestive heart failure and asymptomatic ventricular arrhythmia. N Engl J Med 333:77-82, 1995

50. Hohnloser SH, Klingenheben T, Singh BN: Amiodarone-associated proarrhythmic effects. A review with special reference to torsade de pointes tachycardia. Ann Intern Med 121:529-535, 1994

51. Chiale PA, Halpern MS, Nau GJ, Tambussi AM, Przybylski J, Lazzari JO, Elizari MV, Rosenbaum MB: Efficacy of amiodarone during long-term treatment of malignant ventricular arrhythmias in patients with chronic chagasic myocarditis. Am Heart J 107:656-665, 1984

52. Rosenbaum MB, Chiale PA, Haedo A, Lazzari JO, Elizari MV: Ten years of experience with amiodarone. Am Heart J 106:957-964, 1983

53. Heger JJ, Prystowsky EN, Jackman WM, Naccarelli GV, Warfel KA, Rinkenberger RL, Zipes DP: Clinical efficacy and electrophysiology during long-term therapy for recurrent ventricular tachycardia or ventricular fibrillation. N Engl J Med 305:539-545, 1981

54. Sobol SM, Rakita L: Pneumonitis and pulmonary fibrosis associated with amiodarone treatment: a possible complication of a new antiarrhythmic drug. Circulation 65:819-824, 1982

55. Chezalviel-Guilbert F, Davy JM, Poirier JM, Weissenburger J: Mexiletine antagonizes effects of sotalol on QT interval duration and its proarrhythmic effects in a canine model of torsade de pointes. J Am Coll Cardiol 26:787-792, 1995

56. Shimizu W, Antzelevitch C: Sodium channel block with mexiletine is effective in reducing dispersion of repolarization and preventing torsade des pointes in LQT2 and LQT3 models of the long-QT syndrome. Circulation 96:2038-2047, 1997

57. Chiale PA, Rosenbaum MB, Elizari MV, Hjalmarson A, Magnusson Y, Wallukat G, Hoebeke J: High prevalence of antibodies against beta 1- and beta 2-adrenoceptors in patients with primary electrical cardiac abnormalities. J Am Coll Cardiol 26:864-869, 1995

58. Ferrari I, Levin MJ, Elizari MV, Rosenbaum MB, Chiale PA: Cholinergic autoantibodies in sinus-node dysfunction (letter). Lancet 350:262-263, 1997

59. de Oliveira SF, Pedrosa RC, Nascimento JH, Campos de Carvalho AC, Masuda MO: Sera from chronic chagasic patients with complex cardiac arrhythmias depress electrogenesis and conduction in isolated rabbit hearts. Circulation 96:2031-2037, 1997

60. Coumel P, Rosengarten MD, Leclercq JF, Attuel P: Role of sympathetic nervous system in non-ischaemic ventricular arrhythmias. Br Heart J 47:137-147, 1982

61. Zipes DP, Maratins JB, Ruffy R et al: Role of the autonomic nervous system in the genesis of ventricular arrhythmias. *In* Frontiers of Cardiac Electrophysiology. Edited by MB Rosenbaum, MV Elizari. Boston, Nijhoff, 1983, pp 522-551

62. Randall WC, Ardell JL: Differential innervation of the heart. *In* Cardiac Electrophysiology and Arrhythmias. Edited by DP Zipes, J Jalife. Orlando, Grune & Stratton, 1985, pp 137-144

63. Gang ES, Oseran DS, Mandel WJ, Peter T: Sinus node electrogram in patients with the hypersensitive carotid sinus syndrome. J Am Coll Cardiol 5:1484-1490, 1985

64. Mueller J, Wallukat G, Dandel M, Bieda H, Spiegelsberger S, Hummel M, Hetzer R: Treatment of idiopathic dilated cardiomyopathy by IgG immunoadsorption (abstract). Circulation 98 Suppl:I-104, 1998

65. Müller J, Wallukat G, Brandes K, Spiegelsberger S, Bieda H, Kupetz W, Hummel M, Hetzer R: Successful therapy of idiopathic dilated cardiomyopathy by IgG immunoadsorption, results of a controlled study (abstract). J Am Coll Cardiol 31 Suppl:67A, 1998

66. Ceremuzynski L, Kleczar E, Krzeminska-Pakula M, Kuch J, Nartowicz E, Smielak-Korombel J, Dyduszynski A, Maciejewicz J, Zaleska T, Lazarczyk-Kedzia E, Motyka J, Pazkowska B, Sczaniecka O, Yusuf S: Effect of amiodarone on mortality after myocardial infarction: a double-blind, placebo-controlled, pilot study. J Am Coll Cardiol 20:1056-1062, 1992

67. Julian DG, Camm AJ, Frangin G, Janse MJ, Munoz A, Schwartz PJ, Simon P, for the European Myocardial Infarct Amiodarone Trial Investigators: Randomised trial of effect of amiodarone on mortality in patients with left-ventricular dysfunction after recent myocardial infarction: EMIAT. Lancet 349:667-674, 1997

68. Cairns JA, Connolly SJ, Roberts R, Gent M, for the Canadian Amiodarone Myocardial Infarction Arrhythmia Trial Investigators: Randomised trial of outcome after myocardial infarction in patients with frequent or repetitive ventricular premature depolarisations: CAMIAT. Lancet 349:675-682, 1997

69. Zipes DP: An overview of arrhythmias and antiarrhythmic approaches. J Cardiovasc Electrophysiol 10:267-271, 1999

70. Moncayo A: Chagas' disease. Division of Control of Tropical Diseases. World Health Organization (printed by Sadag, France), Geneva, 1996

Chapter 9

Surgery and Catheter Ablation for the Treatment of Ventricular Tachycardia in Chagas' Disease

Eduardo Sosa, M.D.,
Mauricio Scanavacca, M.D.,
André d'Avila, M.D.

Chagas' disease is a major health issue for Latin America, where over 16 million people are affected by the disease. In addition, more than 90 million people are exposed to the risk of acquiring the disease. The cardiovascular system can be affected in several distinct ways, one of which is sustained ventricular tachycardia (VT).[1-5] Although the prevalence of VT in chagasic patients is unknown, approximately half the patients at the Heart Institute of the University of São Paulo, Brazil, who undergo electrophysiologic studies because of VT or cardiac arrest have Chagas' disease.[6]

The electrophysiologic mechanism involved in this arrhythmia and its clinical characteristics have been partially elucidated. It consists of a reentrant type VT.[6,7] Frequently, these arrhythmic episodes are concentrated in short periods, creating what is commonly called a "chagasic storm." Rarely, this VT evolves to an incessant form, making treatment extremely difficult. Drug therapy for VT is inefficient for patients in New York Heart Association (NYHA) class III or IV for heart failure, since the recurrence rate is 100% and mortality in the subsequent year is 40%. Although treatment with amiodarone does not prevent VT recurrences (30% a year) for patients in NYHA functional class I or II, sudden death is a rare event in these patients.[8]

From Tentori MC, Segura EL, Hayes DL (eds.) *Arrhythmia Management in Chagas' Disease.* Armonk, NY: Futura Publishing Co., Inc. ©2000.

Myocardial damage occurs in various portions of both ventricles, but the basal inferolateral segment of the left ventricle is the most frequent site of origin of VT in chagasic patients.[9-11] Endocardial mapping techniques show fragmentation on ventricular electrograms and late potentials in sinus rhythm as well as early or continuous diastolic electrical activity during VT systematically arising from that region (Fig. 9-1).

Although restricted to a specific area of the left ventricle, the circuit does not seem to be small. A major fragmentation on left ventricular electrograms can also be registered from electrodes positioned in the coronary sinus (Fig. 9-2) and at the posterior ascending cardiac vein, results suggesting that the VT circuit might involve the epicardial surface of the left ventricle.

Because of the prevalence of Chagas' disease in Latin America,[12] several institutions in many countries are studying arrhythmias in the disease. However, results obtained at those institutions for the treatment of cardiac arrhythmia in patients with the disease are difficult to evaluate for several reasons. The heterogeneous pattern of the disease, its multiple clinical presentations, and the short-term follow-up undertaken in very selected groups of patients make comparison of these results difficult. Moreover, each center individualizes the therapies according to the available treatment possibilities. In doing so, each center tries to justify its own therapeutic options, but fundamental questions related to patient prognosis with one of the several types of treatment are intuitively answered, resulting in limited scientific significance.

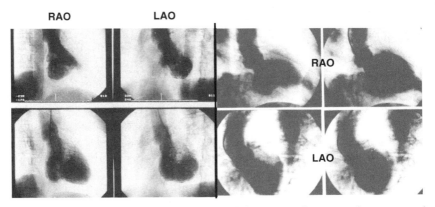

Fig. 9-1. Left and right panels contrast left ventriculograms during systole and diastole in the right (RAO) and left (LAO) anterior oblique projections. In the left panel, an inferolateral aneurysm produces the typical angiographic appearance for a patient with chagasic ventricular tachycardia. Not only the inferolateral aneurysm but also an anteroseptal aneurysm, usually described as a nipple or glove's finger lesion, are seen. The apical aneurysm is a very characteristic lesion and considered by some to be a pathognomonic lesion of Chagas' cardiomyopathy. Although highly prevalent in patients with Chagas' disease, it is rarely the origin of ventricular tachycardia.

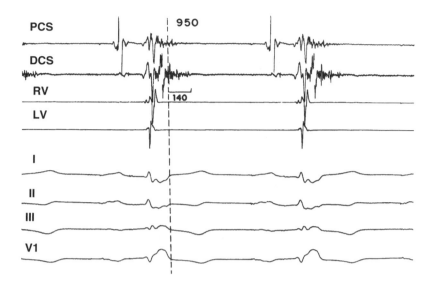

Fig. 9-2. Fractionation on ventricular bipolar electrogram recorded from the proximal and distal pair of electrodes inserted in the coronary sinus during sinus rhythm (cycle length, 950 msec) in a chagasic patient with right bundle branch block. Late potentials are noted for 140 msec after the QRS complex. This finding indicates late activation of viable epicardial myocardium cells. Shown are electrocardiographic leads I, II, III, and V_1. DCS, distal coronary sinus; LV, left ventricle; PCS, proximal coronary sinus; RV, right ventricle.

Because of these limitations, treatment of chagasic VT is generally extrapolated from results obtained in patients with coronary heart disease. However, some differences between these patients are worth noting. Chagasic patients tend to be younger and have a higher left ventricular ejection fraction. It is assumed, therefore, that their prognosis is closely related to VT treatment rather than to progression of the myocardial damage caused by the disease itself.

The objective of this chapter is to review the results of ablative procedures (surgical and catheter ablation) used at our institution to modify, destroy, or isolate segments of the ventricles that are responsible for sustaining VT in chagasic patients. It is important to understand that these procedures were used in a highly selected group of patients with sustained monomorphic VT that was reproducible after programmed ventricular stimulation and well tolerated to allow extensive electrophysiologic mapping.

Surgical Approach

Electrophysiologically Guided Resection

Surgery for chagasic VT began at our institution in 1979. At that time, an apical aneurysm was assumed to be of utmost importance, since it was believed that chagasic VT, like ischemic VT, was related to an anteroapical aneurysm.[9-11]

Programmed electrical stimulation performed in surgery during normothermia allowed induction of stable VT in 14 of 21 patients (67%) in whom epicardial mapping was feasible. The VT site of origin was defined intraoperatively as the site of earliest endocardial activation. Whenever intraoperative mapping was inadequate, a target site was selected on the basis of data obtained during preoperative mapping and their relation to affected left ventricular segments.

Surgical treatment consisted of conventional aneurysmectomy with endocardial or myocardial resection or isolation of a selected area by endocardial resection. (Cryotherapy was not available at our institution at that time.)

Patients were divided into two groups. Group A consisted of 14 patients with left ventricular ejection fraction greater than 40%. Group B consisted of 11 patients with left ventricular ejection fraction of 40% or less. Interestingly, when we compared the site of origin of VT and the position of the aneurysm, VT originated in the inferolateral region of the left ventricle in 11 patients from group A (78%), 9 of whom had large apical aneurysms. In group B, all the patients had apical aneurysms, but only three (27%) had VT related to them. In the remaining eight patients (73%), VT also originated at the inferolateral segment of the left ventricle. When the groups were analyzed together, VT originated in the inferolateral region of the left ventricle in 76% of the patients and in an anteroapical region in 24%. On the basis of these findings, we could assume that for chronic chagasic cardiomyopathy, the inferolateral region of the left ventricle was the most frequent site of VT origin, a conclusion eventually confirmed in other studies (Fig. 9-3).

Programmed ventricular stimulation performed with epicardial wires 2 weeks after surgery did not induce VT in 15 of the patients (60%). Hospital mortality was 20% (5 of 25). On dismissal from the hospital, the survivors were treated with amiodarone; 20% (4 of 20) died within the next 12 months.[9-11]

Anatomically Guided Surgical Approach

A possible cause of the low success rate of surgical treatment arose from histologic analysis of chagasic lesions. Such analyses revealed bundles of diseased myocardial fibers alternating with a large amount of viable myocardium. It was assumed that in this substrate, reentry via normal myocardial fibers was a highly reasonable possibility. It was thus assumed that the success of the procedure depended on destruction of a larger amount of tissue.

Between April 1991 and August 1994, 19 consecutive patients (10 of whom were female; age range, 47 to 68 years) were treated by interpapillary endomyocardial cryoablation. All had basal inferolateral

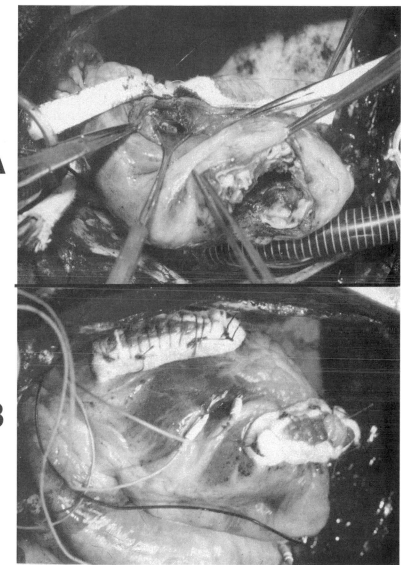

Fig. 9-3. *A,* Resection of both inferior and anterior left ventricular aneurysms in a chagasic patient with ventricular tachycardia (VT). This was the first patient in whom VT persisted after resection of the anterior aneurysm. *B,* Intraoperative mapping localized the earliest activation site in the posteroinferior wall. In our subsequent patients, 76% had VT related to an inferolateral aneurysm, whereas only 24% had VT related to an anteroseptal aneurysm.

akinesia or dyskinesia, and the site of origin of VT was determined according to the earliest endocardial activation shown during preoperative mapping. No operative mapping was done in these patients.[9-11]

After establishment of extracorporeal circulation and hypothermic cardioplegia, the inferolateral region was exposed, and a 2- to 4-cm incision was made between the papillary muscles on the akinetic region perpendicular to the atrioventricular ring. The ventricular wall in this region was usually very thin ($\pm$ 4 mm). Once the left ventricular cavity was exposed, multiple -70°C cryothermic applications were made with a 4-cm probe (Fig. 9-4) until it was assumed that the area was homogeneously destroyed.

In this series, there was no hospital mortality. On the 15th postoperative day, all patients had programmed electrical stimulation, with VT induction in 6 patients (31%). Ten of the patients (53%) were dismissed with a regimen of amiodarone, 200 mg daily, because of frequent premature ventricular beats. In a 24-month follow-up, there were two spontaneous recurrences of VT (10%) and two deaths (one sudden death and one due to heart failure).

Success was similar for both guided and nonguided surgical procedures, but mortality was lower for the latter. A possible reason for

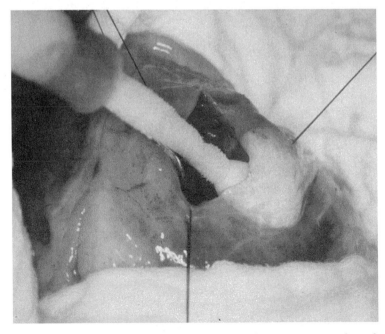

Fig. 9-4. Left ventricular cavity is exposed through an incision in the inferolateral aneurysm. This region usually has a very thin ventricular wall. In some patients, it is even translucent. Multiple cryothermic applications at a temperature of –70°C are performed with a 4-cm probe until it is assumed that the area is homogeneously destroyed.

failure to ablate VT could be the persistence of areas of viable myocardium between sites of cryoablation in regions that could permit reentry. From the surgeon's point of view, the existence of reversible areas close to cryoablation sites was not an acceptable outcome; irreversible and more homogeneous lesions could result in a lower rate of failures. Finally, cryoablation may not be enough to produce transmural lesions.

Catheter Ablation

On the basis of Hartzler's demonstration[13] that VT after myocardial infarction could be ablated with direct current shocks, we decided to test that procedure in chagasic VT. This procedure was first attempted at our institution in 1987 in a patient with VT related to basal inferolateral akinesia of the left ventricle who had preserved left ventricular global contractility. Three direct current shocks of 300 J were delivered at the earliest activation site, and thereafter VT was not inducible. This patient was asymptomatic without antiarrhythmic drugs for 6 years, when he was lost to follow-up. It was then demonstrated that chagasic VT could be ablated with catheters, and new possibilities arose for the treatment of this arrhythmia. Although a few instances of VT could be controlled with endocardial fulguration, general results with this technique were disappointing.[14]

Catheter Ablation With Alcohol

Theoretically, transcoronary catheter ablation of VT offers more possibilities than direct current shock or surgical resection techniques. First, transcoronary administration of iced saline allows us to test whether the selected site is correct. As a result, unnecessary damage caused by directly injecting ethanol can be avoided. Additionally, the lesion created is transmural, preventing the problems related to intramurally or epicardially located reentry circuits. Finally, it seems that although transcoronary ablation produces particularly large lesions, which are significantly more extensive than those created by radiofrequency ablation, they do not reach the dimensions of those created by endocardial resection and do not alter ventricular function.[15,16]

Transcoronary chemical ablation was studied at our center in patients with Chagas' disease, but the results with this technique were disappointing. After two deaths related to complications, the procedure was abandoned as an alternative treatment of VT associated with Chagas' disease. Nevertheless, we agree that this technique has not been given a fair test of its potential.

Radiofrequency Catheter Ablation

The advent of radiofrequency ablation has allowed us to use it as an alternative to treat VT associated with Chagas' disease. From 1991 to 1996, 24 consecutive patients (16 of whom were male; mean age, 53 ± 8 years) had endocardial radiofrequency catheter ablation. In this group of patients, 52 episodes of sustained ventricular tachycardia could be mapped, with a mean of 2.2 episodes per patient. After 26 ± 21 months of follow-up, success (defined as no interruption, no reinduction, and no spontaneous VT recurrence in patients receiving amiodarone, 200 mg/day) was achieved in only 17% of the patients. Although there were no complications, the success rate was disappointing in contrast to our results in patients with VT after myocardial infarction. At that time, we hypothesized that epicardial circuits could explain the poor results of standard endocardial radiofrequency ablation. This thought led us to introduce a novel technique of transthoracic epicardial ablation.

Transthoracic Epicardial Ablation

Data obtained from intraoperative mapping suggest that epicardial circuits are a common finding in postinfarction VT related to the left ventricular inferior wall.[17] In these circumstances, conventional pulses of radiofrequency energy may be less effective. Radiofrequency ablation may fail to abolish these ventricular arrhythmias because the temperature is unlikely to increase to 50°C in deeper tissues, and standard endocardial catheter ablation may fail because of possible epicardial target sites. Interestingly, chagasic VT originates from the left ventricular inferior wall in most patients. One could thus speculate that chagasic VT ablation fails because of epicardial or intramyocardial (or both) reentrant circuits.

To determine whether epicardial circuits are present, analysis of epicardial electrograms is crucial. Until recently, however, epicardial mapping was done only during cardiac surgery and was thus restricted to the operating room. Attempts to map the epicardial surface with a less invasive approach, through thoracoscopy, were soon abandoned, not only because of the need to perform it in the surgical room but also because of difficulty in keeping the catheter stable. Another limitation was restriction of the accessible area for mapping to the anterior ventricular wall. Alternatively, insertion of multipolar catheters into the pulmonary veins may be used to obtain epicardial signs, as previously described. However, mapping is limited by the cardiac anatomy, and the technique is not helpful when the site of origin is not close enough to the epicardial veins.[18,19]

Transthoracic epicardial mapping, a technique introduced by our group in 1996, permits a great deal of epicardial exploration in the electrophysiology laboratory.[20] Briefly, a standard ablation catheter with a 4-mm tip is introduced into the pericardial space by transthoracic epicardial puncture, a procedure similar to that Krikorian and Hancock[21] described for drainage of pericardial effusions. The feasibility and safety of the procedure for VT mapping and ablation have previously been described.

Our current impression is that this technique has increased our ability to treat chagasic VT, and preliminary but encouraging results have been published.[22] In one of these studies, 10 consecutive patients with chronic chagasic cardiomyopathy and VT received epicardial mapping and radiofrequency ablation. Eighteen instances of VT could be mapped (one to four per patient), and 14 of these had an epicardial circuit. Four were interrupted by applications of radiofrequency pulses in the endocardium, guided by epicardial mapping (mean interruption time, 20.1 ± 14 seconds), but all were reinduced. Ten of the remaining 14 were interrupted with radiofrequency pulses in the epicardium, and none was reinduced (Fig. 9-5). One of the patients had a small hemopericardium (about 50 mL), which was drained in the electrophysiology laboratory, and brief pericardial discomfort in three patients was controlled by anti-inflammatory drugs.

This technique has proven to be a safe and effective means of identifying and interrupting epicardial circuits of sustained VT when used to guide radiofrequency epicardial catheter ablation. Thus, it should be incorporated in the electrophysiologic routine of mapping and ablation for patients with VT associated with Chagas' disease in whom epicardial circuits seem to predominate.

Final Comments

Currently, most patients with sustained monomorphic VT associated with chronic chagasic cardiomyopathy are initially considered candidates for radiofrequency endocardial or epicardial ablation. Since ablation is now the treatment of choice (it is needless to wait for VT to be refractory to drug therapy), another option is to find a combination of drugs that prevents inducibility of VT. If this approach fails, the next choice is an implantable cardioverter-defibrillator or surgery. In Brazil, social security does not cover the cost of implantation, and often chagasic patients cannot afford it. Instead, low-risk surgical therapy can be offered to patients with refractory VT.

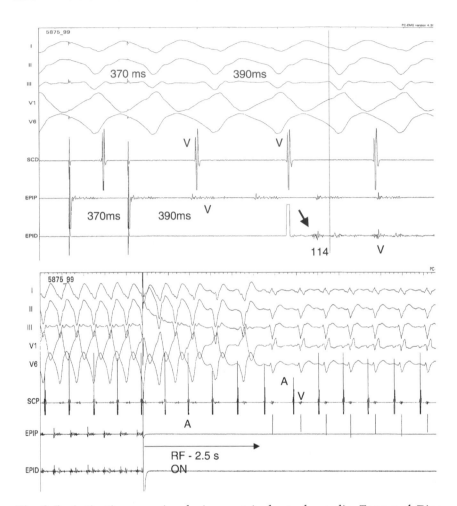

Fig. 9-5. Activation mapping during ventricular tachycardia. *Top panel*, Bipolar pacing from the distal pair of epicardial electrodes (EPID) demonstrates concealed entrainment, with a return cycle identical to the length of the tachycardia cycle. After interruption of ventricular stimulation, an epicardial electrogram (*arrow*) preceding the onset of the QRS complex by 114 msec can be seen in the distal epicardial catheter bipole. *Bottom panel*, An epicardial application of radiofrequency (RF) interrupts ventricular tachycardia within 2.5 seconds and renders it noninducible by ventricular stimulation. Radiofrequency unit set at 60°C. Shown are electrocardiographic leads I, II, III, V_1 and V_6. A, atrial electrogram; EPID, distal epicardial recording site; EPIP, proximal epicardial recording site; SCD, distal coronary sinus; SCP, proximal coronary sinus; V, ventricular electrogram.

References

1. Hagar JM, Rahimtoola SH: Chagas' heart disease. Curr Probl Cardiol 20:825-924, 1995
2. Amorim DS: Chagas' disease. *In* Progress in Cardiology. Vol 8. Edited by PN Yu, JF Goodwin. Philadelphia, Lea & Febiger, 1979, pp 235-279
3. Rosenbaum MB: Chagasic cardiomyopathy. Prog Cardiovasc Dis 7:199-225, 1964
4. Elizari MV, Chiale PA: Cardiac arrhythmias in Chagas' heart disease. J Cardiovasc Electrophysiol 4:596-608, 1993
5. Prata A: Natural history of Chagasic cardiomyopathy. *In* New Approaches in American Trypanosomiasis Research, Scientific Publication 318. Washington, DC, Pan American Health Organization, 1976, p 191
6. Scanavacca M, Sosa E: Electrophysiologic study in chronic Chagas' heart disease. Rev Paul Med 113:841-850, 1995
7. de Paola AA, Horowitz LN, Miyamoto MH, Pinheiro R, Ferreira DF, Terzian AB, Cirenza C, Guiguer N Jr, Portugal OP: Angiographic and electrophysiologic substrates of ventricular tachycardia in chronic Chagasic myocarditis. Am J Cardiol 65:360-363, 1990
8. Scanavacca MI, Sosa EA, Lee JH, Bellotti G, Pileggi F: Empiric therapy with amiodarone in patients with chronic Chagas cardiomyopathy and sustained ventricular tachycardia [Portuguese]. Arq Bras Cardiol 54:367-371, 1990
9. Sosa E, Scanavacca M, Barbero Marcial M, et al: Surgical treatment of cardiac arrhythmias. *In* Eletrofisiologia Clínica e Intervencionista das Arritmias Cardias. Edited by FES Cruz Filho, IG Maia. Rio de Janeiro, Editora Revinter Ltda., 1997, pp 443-455
10. Sosa E, Marcial MB, Pileggi F, Arie S, Scalabrini A, Roma L, Grupi C, Takeshita N, Verginelli G: Ventricular tachycardia–directed surgical treatment. Initial experience [Portuguese]. Arq Bras Cardiol 38:449-454, 1982
11. Sosa EA, Scanavacca M, Marcial MB, Jatene, et al: Terapêutica não-farmacologica das arritmias. *In* SOCESP Cardiologia. Edited by AGMR Souza, A Mansur. São Paulo, Editora Atheneu, 1996, p 922
12. Laranja FS, Dias E, Nobrega G, Miranda A: Chagas' disease; a clinical, epidemiologic, and pathologic study. Circulation 14:1035-1060, 1956
13. Hartzler GO: Electrode catheter ablation of refractory focal ventricular tachycardia. J Am Coll Cardiol 2:1107-1113, 1983
14. Sosa E, Scalabrini A, Rati, et al: Successful catheter ablation of the origin of recurrent ventricular tachycardia in chronic chagasic heart disease. J Electrophysiol 1:58-61, 1987
15. Brugada P, de Swart H, Smeets JL, Wellens HJ: Transcoronary chemical ablation of ventricular tachycardia. Circulation 79:475-482, 1989
16. de Paola AA, Gomes JA, Miyamoto MH, Fo EE: Transcoronary chemical ablation of ventricular tachycardia in chronic chagasic myocarditis. J Am Coll Cardiol 20:480-482, 1992
17. Kaltenbrunner W, Cardinal R, Dubuc M, Shenasa M, Nadeau R, Tremblay G, Vermeulen M, Savard P, Page PL: Epicardial and endocardial mapping of ventricular tachycardia in patients with myocardial infarction. Is the origin of the tachycardia always subendocardially localized? Circulation 84:1058-1071, 1991

18. Arruda M, Chandrasekaran K, Reynolds D, Kugelmass A, Lazzara R, Jackman WM: Idiopathic epicardial outflow tract ventricular tachycardia: implications for RF catheter ablation (abstract). Pacing Clin Electrophysiol 19:611, 1996

19. de Paola AA, Melo WD, Tavora MZ, Martinez EE: Angiographic and electrophysiological substrates for ventricular tachycardia mapping through the coronary veins. Heart 79:59-63, 1998

20. Sosa E, Scanavacca M, d'Avila A, Pilleggi F: A new technique to perform epicardial mapping in the electrophysiology laboratory. J Cardiovasc Electrophysiol 7:531-536, 1996

21. Krikorian JG, Hancock EW: Pericardiocentesis. Am J Med 65:808-814, 1978

22. Sosa E, Scanavacca M, D'Avila A, Piccioni J, Sanchez O, Velarde JL, Silva M, Reolao B: Endocardial and epicardial ablation guided by nonsurgical transthoracic epicardiac mapping to treat recurrent ventricular tachycardia. J Cardiovasc Electrophysiol 9:229-239, 1998

Chapter 10

Use of the Implantable Cardioverter-Defibrillator in Chagas' Disease

Claudio Muratore, M.D.,
Rafael Rabinovich, M.D.

Chagas' disease is restricted to the Latin American continent. It is caused by an intracellular parasite, *Trypanosoma cruzi*. The disease is transmitted mainly through a vector, although it may also be congenital or acquired through blood transfusion. The natural evolution of the disease may lead to chronic chagasic cardiomyopathy, which is known as the world's most frequent chronic myocarditis.

Although no current epidemiologic study in large populations with positive serologic findings has been reported, it is widely accepted on the basis of results of partial studies in selected groups that some clinical manifestations of the disease develop in 40% of the infected population. Of that number, 75% are in the indeterminate stage of the disease, characterized by myocardial fibrosis, and the remaining 25% have evolution to an advanced and irreversible stage, manifested predominantly as congestive heart failure.

The natural history of Chagas' disease and the type of cardiac involvement may vary widely from patient to patient. However, patients who die of myocardial damage during the chronic stage of the disease have complications of this cardiomyopathy, such as adverse hemodynamics associated with ventricular aneurysms, malignant ventricular arrhythmias, severe conduction disorders, heart failure, and pulmonary or systemic thromboembolism. Chronic chagasic cardiomyopathy frequently results in work disability and sudden cardiac death. Because more than 20 million people are affected by Chagas' disease in Latin America, this cardiomyopathy is a very serious health problem.

From Tentori MC, Segura EL, Hayes DL (eds.) *Arrhythmia Management in Chagas' Disease*. Armonk, NY: Futura Publishing Co., Inc. ©2000.

At any stage of the disease, sudden cardiac death can be the cause of death and in some persons may be the first symptom of the disease. Unlike the large body of data related to sudden cardiac death due to coronary artery disease (CAD), the information available to determine the incidence of sudden death of chagasic origin and the related risk factors is extremely limited.[1,2] Ambulatory electrocardiographic monitoring (Holter) has enabled physicians to collect detailed information on chagasic patients during the terminal event. In most cases, ventricular fibrillation (VF) is the cause of death.[3]

Treatment of malignant ventricular arrhythmias in Chagas' disease is difficult. Several studies have demonstrated poor efficacy of antiarrhythmic drugs and a high incidence of toxic effects in patients with Chagas' disease. Because of the pattern of ventricular arrhythmias in chronic chagasic cardiomyopathy, the efficacy and tolerance of antiarrhythmic drugs are difficult to verify.[4-6]

Therapeutic strategies developed over the past few years for sustained ventricular tachycardia (VT) in chronic chagasic cardiomyopathy include testing of serial antiarrhythmic drugs,[7] surgical[8,9] and catheter[10] ablation of the tachycardia circuit, and implantation of cardioverter-defibrillators.[11] Unfortunately, neither randomized studies that allow the comparison of the different procedures nor nonrandomized publications on a large population of patients are available to show which method of treatment is best.

Implantable cardioverter-defibrillators (ICDs) are used in patients with sustained VT and in survivors of sudden cardiac arrest, principally those with CAD. No extensive evaluation of the benefits of ICD therapy has been done in patients with Chagas' disease and malignant ventricular arrhythmias, as evidenced by the very few papers published.

Evaluation Before Cardioverter-Defibrillator Implantation

Additional procedures may be extremely important in the preimplantation evaluation of chagasic patients, because results differ from those in patients who received an ICD for another cause. Each potential patient must be carefully evaluated before the implant procedure to confirm that this therapy is appropriate and that no contraindications are evident. Chagasic patients frequently have atrial and ventricular arrhythmias, sinus node dysfunction, severe conduction disorders, and episodes of VT that require thorough evaluation for determination of the feasibility of ICD implantation and selection of the correct device. Table 10-1 lists the most frequently used complementary tests to evaluate the chagasic patient before the ICD is implanted.

Reversible causes of rhythm disturbances, such as electrolyte and metabolic abnormalities, acute myocardial ischemia, and proarrhythmic effects of antiarrhythmic drugs, must be ruled out. Two-dimen-

Table 10-1.
Evaluation Before Cardioverter-Defibrillator Implantation in Patients With
Chronic Chagasic Cardiomyopathy

Examination for reversible causes of arrhythmia
Echocardiography
Coronary arteriography and left ventriculography
Exercise stress testing
Radioisotopic ventriculography
Ambulatory electrocardiographic monitoring
Electrophysiologic study

---

sional echocardiography is an important noninvasive procedure that helps to determine ventricular function and detect wall motion abnormalities. We suggest that all patients have cardiac catheterization, including coronary angiography and ventriculography. Undoubtedly, the information obtained from this test is essential to define any CAD, evaluate the hemodynamics associated with ventricular aneurysms, and identify valvular disease. All these conditions may have prognostic implications.

Exercise testing provides important information on maximum heart rate, chronotropic response, and possible exercise-induced arrhythmias or ischemia. Such additional information can be used to optimize ICD programming.

Ambulatory electrocardiographic monitoring may identify nonsustained VT and correlation with other supraventricular arrhythmias, such as atrial fibrillation. Moreover, bradycardia or other chronic or paroxysmal tachyarrhythmias may affect the choice of the most appropriate ICD. If a patient requires cardiac pacing or has paroxysmal atrial fibrillation, a dual-chamber ICD should be considered.

In our daily practice, an electrophysiologic study is done in all patients for whom an ICD is likely to be indicated. It is important to evaluate different morphologic types of induced VT and their response to ventricular overdrive stimulation. Patients with Chagas' cardiomyopathy, unlike patients with CAD, are likely to have more than one morphologic form of VT or possibly some polymorphic forms.

Clinical Characteristics of Patients With Chagasic Cardiomyopathy

The clinical characteristics of the chagasic patients receiving ICD therapy are similar to those in patients with CAD, except for a higher prevalence of women with Chagas' disease (Table 10-2). This difference might be explained by the fact that the disease is an endemic parasitic infection that affects both sexes indiscriminately. Some characteristics,

Table 10-2.
Clinical Characteristics in 23 Patients With Chagas' Cardiomyopathy

Patient	Age, yr	Sex	NYHA	AF	Pacemaker	Arrhythmia index	EF, %
1	66	M	II			VT	31
2	72	M	I			VT	39
3	58	M	I			VT	45
4	65	M	II			VT	23
5	62	F	II			VT	50
6	59	M	I			VT	33
7	50	F	I			VT	37
8	48	M	0			SCD	28
9	53	F	II			SCD	31
10	60	F	I			SCD	20
11	63	F	III			VT	27
12	65	F	II	Yes		VT	20
13	55	F	II			VT	28
14	62	M	II		Yes	VT	23
15	66	M	III		Yes	VT	47
16	64	M	II	Yes		VT	40
17	66	F	I			VT	35
18	60	M	0			VT	33
19	65	F	II		Yes	VT	31
20	72	F	I			VT	29
21	55	M	II			VT	21
22	40	M	0			VT	50
23	64	M	I			VT	35

AF, atrial fibrillation; EF, ejection fraction; F, female; M, male; NYHA, New York Heart Association functional class; SCD, sudden cardiac arrest; VT, ventricular tachycardia.

such as age, functional class, left ventricular ejection fraction, and arrhythmia index, are similar in both groups.

Most patients seek medical attention after an episode of sustained VT or aborted sudden cardiac arrest. Patients who receive an ICD belong to a highly select group, because the disease prevails in low income populations with limited access to institutions that can provide ICD therapy. The indications for an ICD include lack of clinical response to antiarrhythmic drugs and noninducibility during the initial electrophysiologic study. Because the incidence of sudden cardiac death is high in this population, determining high-risk predictive variables, such as nonsustained VT associated with left ventricular dysfunction, is of interest when an ICD is prescribed prophylactically.

Amiodarone is the antiarrhythmic drug of choice during programmed ventricular stimulation. In our practice, amiodarone is widely prescribed for both atrial and ventricular arrhythmias. Ventricular premature contractions are commonly associated with Chagas' disease. Typically, the patient undergoing evaluation because of an episode of VT has already been treated with amiodarone.

Atrial arrhythmias, particularly atrial fibrillation, occur in 20% to 25% of patients. The history of such rhythm disturbances is relevant to selection and programming of the ICD and to determination of antiarrhythmic management. It is also important to know the chronotropic function, assessed during preimplantation procedures through the stress test and Holter monitoring. Sinus node dysfunction is said to occur in 15% of chagasic patients. Given the high incidence of conduction disorders and sinus node dysfunction, a significant subset of the chagasic population requires permanent antibradycardia support. In our country, Chagas' disease is one of the major conditions that require a permanent pacemaker. In our experience, the need for permanent pacing increased during follow-up, probably because of the use of antiarrhythmic drugs and chagasic involvement of the conduction system.

Chagas' disease and CAD are infrequently associated. We have detected CAD in only one of our patients, a 5% incidence. Our belief is that this association may increase in the future because chagasic patients, mainly male, are migrating, particularly to larger cities, looking for better working conditions. This is already being observed in our country.

Clinical Outcome
of Cardioverter-Defibrillator Implantation

Twenty-one chagasic patients with an ICD were followed up for a mean of 31 ± 22 months (range, 1 to 61 months).[12] At each visit, the status of the sensing and pacing circuit was verified and the high-voltage circuit monitored through evaluation of the impedance of the most recently delivered shock. All therapeutic events were stored in the memory and registered through the printer or recorded on a disk.

In our experience, episodes of malignant ventricular arrhythmia are much more frequent in chagasic patients than in those with other types of underlying heart disease. All our patients had adequate therapy, prompted by VT or VF episodes, delivered by the ICD. Antiarrhythmic drugs were frequently needed during follow-up because of recurrences of VT or VF that required electric shock therapy. Amiodarone was prescribed for 71% of our patients during follow-up.

In one-third of our population, electrical storm developed, defined as repetitive episodes of VT or VF requiring many discharges of the device in a short period. We do not know the exact reasons for the higher incidence of this pattern in patients with Chagas' disease. The high density of ventricular arrhythmia usually found in this population may trigger sustained arrhythmias. On the other hand, modulating factors, such as the neurovegetative alterations typical of this disease, might modify the electrophysiologic substrate.

No data are available on the clinical management of patients with electrical storm, and treatment is generally empirical. Our practice is to admit all patients to an intensive care unit for monitoring and evaluation of reversible causes of triggering and for implementation of antiarrhythmic drug therapy. Beta-blockers have not produced satisfactory results in chagasic patients. In our practice, we have controlled the electrical storms by continuous infusion of isoproterenol until the heart rate exceeds 90 bpm. Another option is to program the ICD to a lower pacing rate of 100 to 110 bpm to overdrive the heart rate. This approach supports the neurovegetative dysfunction hypothesis that has been suggested in these patients. If the patient has not been receiving an antiarrhythmic drug, we consider amiodarone either alone or with mexiletine.

How Often Do We Need to Pace?

Permanent pacing is frequently needed in chagasic patients. As previously noted, causes of bradyarrhythmias include sinus node dysfunction, advanced interventricular conduction disorders, atrioventricular block, and use of antiarrhythmic drugs. Cardiac pacing was required to maintain a stable cardiac rhythm in 26% of our patients.

Complications

The most frequent complication was inappropriate shock. One-fourth of our patients received spurious shocks when supraventricular arrhythmias were detected. This rate is similar to that reported in typical ICD populations. All our patients received a single-chamber ICD. This type of device does not differentiate well between supraventricular and ventricular arrhythmias. We can program only the onset and stability features in such a device. New dual-chamber devices will undoubtedly decrease inappropriate shocks.

Mortality

Four deaths occurred during follow-up. Three were due to heart failure in the terminal phase of the illness, and one death was due to pulmonary thromboembolism. Drug treatment of cardiac failure in chagasic patients was not different from conventional treatment in patients with ischemic cardiomyopathy. It included the use of digitalis, angiotensin-converting enzyme inhibitors, diuretics, and beta-blockers (atenolol, carvedilol) if tolerated. Neither sudden cardiac death nor surgical mortality has occurred in our patients receiving ICD therapy.

Comparison Between
Patients With Chagas' Disease and Patients
With Coronary Artery Disease

The factors tested during ICD implantation were similar to those used for patients with CAD.[11] The ventricular pacing and defibrillation thresholds determined during implantation were comparable in groups of patients with Chagas' disease and CAD[11] (Fig. 10-1). In both populations, 74% of patients had an ICD with monophasic shock delivery, which could account for the relatively high defibrillation thresholds. Another reason is that all patients were taking amiodarone at the time of implantation, and this drug may increase defibrillation thresholds.

We did not find any significant difference in the detected number or rate of spontaneous episodes of VT and VF in relation to the therapeutic shocks delivered by the device during follow-up. Moreover, the effectiveness of antitachycardia pacing was similar in both populations (Fig. 10-2). We observed a greater number of episodes of VT in patients with Chagas' cardiomyopathy, although this trend did not reach statistical significance, probably because the population studied was small. These observations suggest that third-generation ICDs offer similar advantages in management whether VT or VF results from Chagas' disease or from CAD. Because of the greater likelihood of arrhythmic episodes in chagasic patients, it will be interesting to further investigate the effect of ICD systems with options of programmable ventricular overdrive stimulation on diminishing the frequency of sustained or nonsustained ventricular arrhythmias.

Time of First
Implantable Cardioverter-Defibrillator Shock

The time of the first ICD shock and its relationship to mortality have been reported in patients with CAD. Patients with Chagas' cardiomyopathy seem to be more prone than patients with CAD to the development of arrhythmic events in the first months after implantation.[13] In our experience, 55% of patients with Chagas' cardiomyopathy and 14% of patients with CAD received an appropriate shock from the ICD in the first month of follow-up (Fig. 10-3). It has not been possible to establish causes for these differences. We do not think that they can be attributed to the use of antiarrhythmic drugs, such as amiodarone, since drug administration did not differ between the two populations. Impairment of the left ventricular ejection fraction has been identified as an independent clinical predictor of shock occurrence.[14-16] In the population studied, although the left ventricular ejection fraction was similarly depressed in both groups, chagasic patients received more shocks than the patients with CAD. The cumulative incidence of shocks

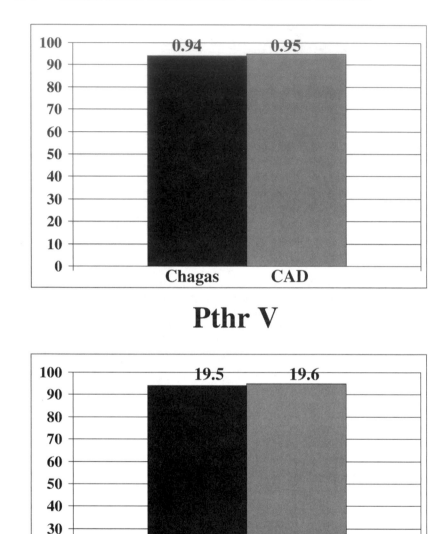

Pthr V

DFT J

Fig. 10-1. Pacing threshold (Pthr) (*top*) and defibrillation threshold (DFT; monophasic wave) (*bottom*) determined during cardioverter-defibrillator implantation in patients with Chagas' cardiomyopathy (Chagas) and patients with coronary artery disease (CAD). J, Joules; V, millivolts.

VT Detection and Therapy

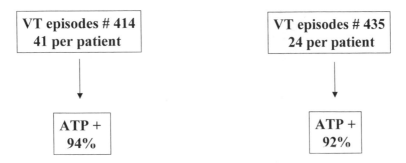

Chagas' disease (n 10)
Follow-up x 19 months

VT episodes # 414
41 per patient

ATP +
94%

CAD (n 18)
Follow-up x 21 months

VT episodes # 435
24 per patient

ATP +
92%

Fig. 10-2. Implantable cardioverter-defibrillator data log in patients with Chagas' disease and patients with coronary artery disease (CAD) analyzed for detection of ventricular tachycardia (VT) and effectiveness of antitachycardia pacing (ATP). No statistically significant differences were observed. ATP +, successful antitachycardia pacing.

per patient within 1, 2, 3, and 6 months after implantation is illustrated in Fig. 10-4. The highest incidence of shock events occurred within the first month.

Even though the incidences of first appropriate shock differed significantly between patients with Chagas' cardiomyopathy and those with CAD, total mortality in patients who received shocks was similar in both groups. Nevertheless, we found that the impact of the first shock and the time the deaths were reported differed between the groups. The time that elapsed between the first shock and death was significantly longer in patients with Chagas' cardiomyopathy than in patients with CAD.

Circadian Rhythm
of Sustained Ventricular Tachyarrhythmias

Circadian variation in spontaneous episodes of VT or VF has been demonstrated in patients with CAD.[17,18] The ICD event recording has become a major means of accurately assessing circadian variation. In patients with CAD, a morning peak and second smaller afternoon peak have been linked to the incidences of both sudden cardiac death and sustained VT.

N° Pt

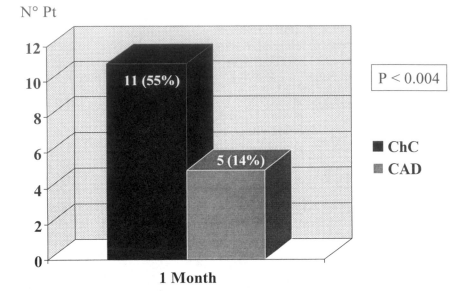

Fig. 10-3. Incidence of implantable cardioverter-defibrillator shocks at 1 month. A statistically significant difference was observed between the two groups. CAD, coronary artery disease; ChC, Chagas' cardiomyopathy.

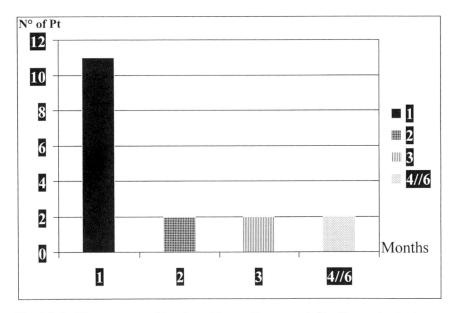

Fig. 10-4. Time course of implantable cardioverter-defibrillator shocks in patients with Chagas' cardiomyopathy. Most of the shocks occurred within the first month.

Circadian rhythm of malignant ventricular arrhythmias in chagasic patients seems to be different from that in patients with CAD. We recently presented our experience in the evaluation of VT or VF circadian rhythm in chagasic patients by comparing them with patients who had CAD.[19] In the population studied, we found that the incidence of arrhythmic events was significantly higher in the morning than in other time periods (Fig. 10-5). Sixty percent of VT episodes occurred in that period, the highest concentration being between 8:00 A.M. and 10:00 A.M. (Fig.10-6). In patients with Chagas' cardiomyopathy, the afternoon peak does not appear, and the reason for this difference remains unknown. The distribution of VF episodes in the four periods analyzed revealed no differences in patterns.

We believe that multiple factors can influence the variations of the "arrhythmic genesis" of chagasic disease. Different hypotheses have been proposed to account for the different behavior of the arrhythmias, including degenerative alterations of cardiac and peripheral nerve plexes and neurovegetative dysfunction.[20,21]

Several authors[20,22,23] have investigated the chagasic lesions, including demyelinating injuries in chagasic models. Such lesions were observed in different organs and tissues, including the nervous plexus of the heart and peripheral organs. Parasympathetic dysfunction and a reduction in sympathetic responsiveness are common features of the disease. Spectral analysis of heart rate variability in patients with Chagas' disease was analyzed by Guzzetti et al.[24] They found alterations in spectral indices of heart rate variability, which may represent markers of neural regulatory dysfunction in both sympathetic and parasympa-

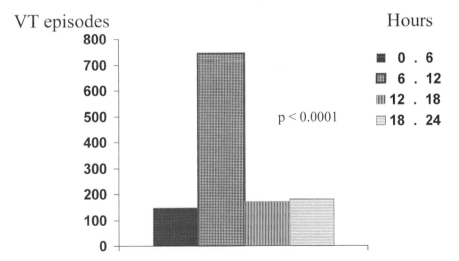

Fig. 10-5. Distribution of ventricular tachycardia (VT) during four portions of the day. The circadian pattern was characterized by a marked peak between 6 A.M. and noon (60% of all VT episodes). The number of events is shown on the y-axis.

VT episodes

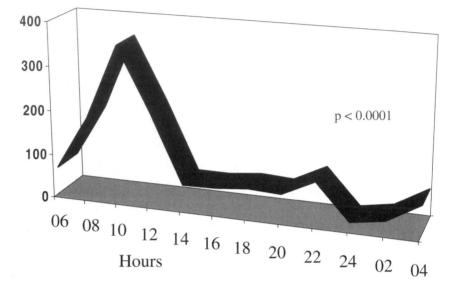

Fig. 10-6. Circadian variation of ventricular tachycardia (VT). There was a statistically significant difference in the circadian rhythm of VT between patients with Chagas' cardiomyopathy and those with coronary artery disease, with a peak between 8 and 10 A.M. in the patients with Chagas' disease. The number of VT episodes is noted on the y-axis.

thetic systems. It is possible that in patients with Chagas' cardiomyopathy, similar impairment of autonomic nervous tone has a prominent place in the genesis of ventricular arrhythmias. Other factors, such as myocardial ischemia, myocardial infarction, and abnormal platelet aggregability and coronary blood flow, have not been demonstrated in Chagas' disease.

Conclusions

Within the past 18 years, there has been a tremendous growth in the use of ICDs. Currently, most patients who receive this device are in the highest risk group, having experienced sudden cardiac arrest or sustained VT. Some trials have suggested that ICD implantation should be the treatment of choice in this high-risk group. At present, patients with sustained VT or aborted sudden cardiac arrest and Chagas' cardiomyopathy seem to receive the same benefits of ICD therapy as patients with CAD. Because of low peri-implant mortality and morbidity with transvenous lead systems, ICD implantation is a logical and cost-effective form of therapy.

References

1. González J, Questa U, Medina F, Posse R: Muerte súbita cardíaca y enfermedad de Chagas. In El Tratamiento de las Arritmias Ventriculares en la Miocarditis Chagásica. Edited by R Posse, T González, A Lapuente, N Barro. Buenos Aires, Ganglionone Estab Gráf, 1983
2. Moleiro F, Mendoza I: 15 year prospective study in chronic Chagas cardiomyopathy (abstract). Circulation 58:II-32, 1978
3. Mendoza I: Muerte súbita y enfermedad de Chagas. Revista Federación Argentina de Cardiología 17:222-223, 1988
4. Mendoza I, Camardo J, Moleiro F, Castellanos A, Medina V, Gomez J, Acquatella H, Casal H, Tortoledo F, Puigbo J: Sustained ventricular tachycardia in chronic chagasic myocarditis: electrophysiologic and pharmacologic characteristics. Am J Cardiol 57:423-427, 1986
5. Mendoza I, Moleiro F, Posse R, et al: Validez de un protocolo de estudio para el tratamiento de las arritmias ventriculares en la miocarditis crónica chagásica. Utilidad de la mexiletine. Rev Latina Cardiol 3:505-511, 1982
6. Chiale PA, Halpern MS, Nau GJ, Tambussi AM, Przybylski J, Lazzari JO, Elizari MV, Rosenbaum MB: Efficacy of amiodarone during long-term treatment of malignant ventricular arrhythmias in patients with chronic chagasic myocarditis. Am Heart J 107:656-665, 1984
7. Giniger AG, Retyk EO, Laino RA, Sananes EG, Lapuente AR: Ventricular tachycardia in Chagas' disease. Am J Cardiol 70:459-462, 1992
8. Milei J, Pesce R, Valero E, Muratore C, Beigelman R, Ferrans VJ: Electrophysiologic-structural correlations in chagasic aneurysms causing malignant arrhythmias. Int J Cardiol 32:65-73, 1991
9. Muratore C, Valero E, Pesce R, Weinschelbaum E, Favaloro R: Tratamiento quirúrgico de la taquicardia ventricular en la miocardiopatía chagásica crónica. Rev Arg de Cardiología 55 Suppl:S16, 1987
10. Sosa E, Scanavacca M, D'Avila A, Bellotti G, Pilleggi F: Radiofrequency catheter ablation of ventricular tachycardia guided by nonsurgical epicardial mapping in chronic Chagasic heart disease. Pacing Clin Electrophysiol 22:128-130, 1999
11. Muratore C, Rabinovich R, Iglesias R, Gonzalez M, Daru V, Liprandi AS: Implantable cardioverter defibrillators in patients with Chagas' disease: are they different from patients with coronary disease? Pacing Clin Electrophysiol 20:194-197, 1997
12. Muratore C, Rabinovich R, Iglesias R, et al: Chagas' cardiomyopathy. Usefulness of implantable cardioverter defibrillator devices in the treatment of malignant ventricular arrhythmias (abstract). J Am Coll Cardiol 31 Suppl:308-C, 1998
13. Rabinovich R, Muratore C, Iglesias R, Gonzalez M, Daru V, Valentino M, Liprandi AS, Luceri R: Time to first shock in implantable cardioverter defibrillator (ICD) patients with Chagas cardiomyopathy. Pacing Clin Electrophysiol 22:202-205, 1999
14. Fogoros RN, Elson JJ, Bonnet CA: Actuarial incidence and pattern of occurrence of shocks following implantation of the automatic implantable cardioverter defibrillator. Pacing Clin Electrophysiol 12:1465-1473, 1989
15. Myerburg RJ, Luceri RM, Thurer R, Cooper DK, Zaman L, Interian A, Fernandez P, Cox M, Glicksman F, Castellanos A: Time to first shock and

clinical outcome in patients receiving an automatic implantable cardi-overter-defibrillator. J Am Coll Cardiol 14:508-514, 1989

16. Dolack GL, for the CASCADE Investigators: Clinical predictors of implantable cardioverter-defibrillator shocks (results of the CASCADE trial). Am J Cardiol 73:237-241, 1994

17. Tofler GH, Gebara OC, Mittleman MA, Taylor P, Siegel W, Venditti FJ Jr, Rasmussen CA, Muller JE, for the CPI Investigators: Morning peak in ventricular tachyarrhythmias detected by time of implantable cardioverter/defibrillator therapy. Circulation 92:1203-1208, 1995

18. Willich SN, Levy D, Rocco MB, Tofler GH, Stone PH, Muller JE: Circadian variation in the incidence of sudden cardiac death in the Framingham Heart Study population. Am J Cardiol 60:801-806, 1987

19. Rabinovich R, Muratore C, Gonzalez M, Iglesias R, Sosa Liprandi A, Luceri R: Circadian variation of ventricular arrhythmias in patients with Chagas cardiomyopathy (abstract). Pacing Clin Electrophysiol 20:1163, 1997

20. Mott KE, Hagstrom JWC: The pathologic lesions of the cardiac autonomic nervous system in chronic Chagas' myocarditis. Circulation 31:273-286, 1965

21. Marin-Neto JA, Maciel BC, Gallo Junior L, Junqueira Junior LF, Amorim DS: Effect of parasympathetic impairment on the haemodynamic response to handgrip in Chagas's heart disease. Br Heart J 55:204-210, 1986

22. Said G, Joskowicz M, Barreira AA, Eisen H: Neuropathy associated with experimental Chagas' disease. Ann Neurol 18:676-683, 1985

23. Molina HA, Cardoni RL, Rimoldi MT: The neuromuscular pathology of experimental Chagas' disease. J Neurol Sci 81:287-300, 1987

24. Guzzetti S, Iosa D, Pecis M, Bonura L, Prosdocimi M, Malliani A: Impaired heart rate variability in patients with chronic Chagas' disease. Am Heart J 121:1727-1734, 1991

Bradyarrhythmias in Chagasic Cardiomyopathy

Claudio de Zuloaga, M.D.

In 1909, Carlos Chagas first showed conduction disturbances and arrhythmias in patients with trypanosomiasis, which he had previously discovered.[1] At the time, he observed a high incidence rate of intraventricular conduction abnormalities, among which right bundle branch block (RBBB) and a variety of ventricular arrhythmias prevailed. The specific involvement of the conduction system and the specific histologic alterations that characterize the disease were subsequently described by different authors. It has been established that regardless of specific histologic alterations, the major jeopardy to the intraventricular conduction system is that every structure from the sinoatrial node to the Purkinje fibers may be affected.

The conduction abnormalities are a result of diffuse lesions with fibrous and fatty replacement throughout the whole system, the finding of focal changes being rather exceptional. Other clinical manifestations—cardiac dilatation and hemodynamic failure—are always preceded by conduction disturbances, which in turn are late symptoms and may take over 20 years to become apparent.[2,3] The extremely high incidence of intraventricular conduction disorders, such as RBBB, associated with left anterior fascicular block allows strong suspicion of the disease, even when the discovery is a single electrocardiographic finding in patients from endemic areas. Conversely, left bundle branch block (LBBB) and isolated hemifascicular blocks are rare.[4]

In summary, the atrioventricular (AV) conduction system is diffusely involved, as shown by the variety of disturbances encountered in patients with Chagas' disease. In addition to compromise of the sinoatrial node, AV nodal and intraventricular conduction system

From Tentori MC, Segura EL, Hayes DL (eds.) *Arrhythmia Management in Chagas' Disease.* Armonk, NY: Futura Publishing Co., Inc. ©2000.

blocks are frequently observed in the final stages of the disease. Two phases—acute and chronic—are distinguished in Chagas' disease, and most conduction abnormalities are found in the latter.

Acute Phase of Chagas' Myocarditis

In this stage, diffuse inflammatory changes are seen throughout the conduction system. The conducting fibers are characteristically separated by edema and mononuclear infiltrate, and inflammatory tissue with lymphocytes and plasma cells has also been described.[5] However, the conduction disturbances are far less common than myocardial involvement, with cavity dilatation and congestive heart failure that hardly ever cause death.

Among the few patients with conduction abnormalities, some atrial and ventricular arrhythmias have been observed—from atrial fibrillation to polymorphic ventricular premature beats with tachycardia or ventricular fibrillation. Malignant arrhythmias are unusual in this stage of Chagas' disease. Therefore, the disturbances may be completely unnoticed by the patients. There are minimal and nonspecific changes in the ST segment and the T wave, a decrease in QRS voltage, and a mild lengthening of the PR interval at the expense of the intranodal conduction.[4] This modification is not related to any of the chronic lesions and cannot be regarded as a prognostic indicator. Laranja et al.,[4] Andrade et al.,[5] and Rosenbaum[2] have shown that significant electrocardiographic (ECG) alterations, such as bundle branch block and complete AV block, portend a poor prognosis when detected at this stage and are often associated with a fatal outcome. These authors have also emphasized that more than 85% of patients who die during the acute phase of Chagas' disease have ECG alterations, whereas these abnormalities are seldom found in asymptomatic patients (37.7%).

Chronic Phase of Chagas' Myocarditis

The most diverse variety of ECG alterations can be noted in the chronic stage of Chagas' disease. Chagas' disease may result in multiple conduction system disturbances in the same patient. How much time is required for the ECG tracings to depict the chronic lesions of the conduction system after the acute infection varies greatly from one patient to another, but the period is usually long.

Anatomically, global dilatation of the heart just like that in an idiopathic cardiomyopathy can occur. Apical aneurysms that can trigger malignant ventricular arrhythmias are not unusual.

Histologically, diffuse and generalized changes are found in the entire conduction system, with fragmentation of the conduction fibers, focal proliferation of histiocytes and lymphocytes, and fibrous and fatty infiltrate alternating with healthy tissue.[6] Complete disruption of the conduction tissue by a single lesion is seldom seen.

Sinoatrial Node

Involvement of the sinoatrial node in Chagas' disease consists of a chronic mononuclear inflammatory infiltrate with atrophy, myocytolysis and necrosis of the specialized fibers, and fatty and fibrous replacement of the nodal tissue.[7] Undoubtedly, this lesion gives rise to a definite alteration of sinus node function.

The real incidence of sinus node dysfunction (SND) in chronic Chagas' cardiomyopathy (CChC) remains controversial because minor abnormalities of sinus node function may not be detected clinically. Hernández-Pieretti et al.[8] found clear disturbances of the sinoatrial node in 15 of 300 patients (5%) with chronic Chagas' disease. In only one-third of these patients was SND an isolated feature without other disorders. In accordance with these findings, Andrade et al.[9] noted a 10% incidence rate of SND in a much smaller series (11 patients). Thus, these alterations could be overlooked if not purposely sought out by specific tests.

Thery et al.[10] found that in patients with a lesion in the sinoatrial node, a suitable sinus rhythm can be maintained even with only 10% of normal (undamaged) cells. This finding probably explains why there is very little clinical evidence of SND in CChC even though this structure is almost always affected by the disease. The underlying cause of the clinical manifestations of SND is more likely to be either sinoatrial block or an association between sinoatrial block and an autonomic disorder rather than genuine loss of automatic cells of the sinoatrial node.

Damage to the intracardiac autonomic nervous system in CChC is no doubt a major factor in the appearance of bradycardia. This involvement is present in both the acute and the chronic phases, causing injury from neurophagia, disintegration of the axis cylinders, and vacuolization of the nerve cells.[11] Köberle[12] showed that neuropathic toxins elaborated by dead parasites are responsible for the neurologic damage. Autonomic dysfunction expressed by reduced baroflex bradycardia and impaired efferent parasympathetic activity caused by intrinsic neuroganglionic lesions have also been pointed out.[13,14]

In brief, the clinical manifestations of SND in CChC are the result of a combination of autonomic damage and organic involvement of the sinoatrial node. On the other hand, various forms of ECG disorders may be depicted in SND. However, sinus bradycardia and sinoatrial block with junctional escape rhythms are more often observed. Nevertheless, sinoatrial blocks without significant bradycardia can be found (Fig. 11-1).

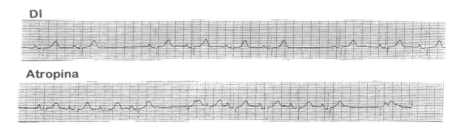

Fig. 11-1. Electrocardiographic findings in a patient with Chagas' cardiomyopathy. *Upper panel*, Baseline recording shows episodes of sinoatrial block without evidence of bradycardia. *Lower panel*, Administration of atropine produces a slight shortening of the sinus cycle, persistence of sinoatrial block, and a junctional beat after sinoatrial block.

Atrioventricular Node

Severe damage to the AV node is extremely rare in CChC. Elizari et al.[15] showed that involvement of the AV node is an unusual event in this disease and that complete AV block with narrow QRS complex is exceptional. Microscopically, lymphocytes, macrophages, and plasma cells are scattered around the node,[5] with significant mononuclear infiltration at the periphery and small foci of healthy tissue in the center.[16] The inflammatory and degenerative lesions of the node become more apparent in the penetrating portion.[5] This particular distribution allows conduction to continue undisrupted at this level without producing complete AV block despite the common occurrence and magnitude of the histologic involvement.

According to our experience, however, intranodal and associated intraventricular conduction disturbances are not uncommon when electrophysiologic assessment of the conduction system is performed. Although not critical, diffuse involvement of the AV node can be suspected during an electrophysiologic study if the AH interval is normal despite prolongation of the functional and effective refractory periods during delivery of premature atrial stimuli.

Bundle of His

From the functional point of view, the His bundle is probably the least compromised structure in CChC, since most complete AV blocks are infra-His.[15] Histologic studies show that the injuries occur almost exclusively in the right half of the His bundle, with the left half usually spared. This distribution is consistent with involvement of the rest of the intraventricular conduction system, in which the right branch is always histologically more affected than the left one. The His bundle is seldom completely disrupted, and the histologic findings are the same as those in other portions of the conduction system: diffuse fibrosis, muscular atrophy, and focal lymphocytic and fatty infiltration.[5]

More often than not, invasive procedures are required to detect disorders in the His bundle. Rapid atrial pacing can at times demonstrate intra-His disturbances that remain completely unnoticed in basal conditions. This latent disorder may trigger syncope. Whether these changes would evolve to complete AV block is uncertain, so that determining a prognosis on the basis of these findings is difficult in patients without symptoms. As in other cardiomyopathies, the predictive value of intra-His conduction abnormalities unmasked during rapid atrial pacing remains obscure.

Left and Right Bundle Branches

Involvement at this level of the conduction system is responsible for most clinically significant bradyarrhythmias and is the major feature to be considered during assessment of the evolution in patients with CChC.

RBBB is the earliest and most frequent finding in patients infected with *Trypanosoma cruzi*. Rosenbaum and Alvarez[17] were among the first researchers to define the incidence of RBBB. They demonstrated RBBB in 55.7% of patients with this disease. The anterior division of the left bundle branch is often involved in patients with CChC, but this is rarely an isolated event and is almost always associated with RBBB. Conduction through the left bundle branch is uncommon. The incidence rate of LBBB (2%) is far lower than that of RBBB.[4]

The higher incidence of RBBB over LBBB has given rise to several postulations. Rosenbaum et al.[18] supported the notion that the incidence is different because chronic myocarditis is actually a panmyocarditis that randomly involves different areas of the heart. These investigators thought that the right bundle branch is more often affected because it is longer and thinner and has a predominantly intramyocardial course. On the other hand, the left branch is short and wide and has a subepicardial course, which make it less vulnerable to these injuries. Andrade et al.[5] suggested otherwise on the basis of histologic findings in 25 patients who died of Chagas' disease, claiming that the injuries to the right and left branches are due to the special predilection of CChC for the conduction system, with a remarkable trend to affect the right bundle.

The incidence of left posterior hemiblock and RBBB is lower, but this combination is a good indicator of severe involvement of the intraventricular conduction system. It is common knowledge that the interval of intraventricular conduction in these patients often exceeds 90 msec. This association suggests that major damage exists in these branches and that intraventricular conduction is almost exclusively provided by the anterior divisions. Reliance on a monofascicular mode of intraventricular conduction portends a poor prognosis because of the frequent involvement of the anterior division in CChC. Paroxysmal AV block is common in these patients, and it often evolves rapidly to complete AV block.

In Figure 11-2, the instability of this kind of conduction can be noted in a patient with RBBB, left posterior hemiblock, and 1:1 AV conduction in whom complete AV block suddenly occurred during an electrophysiologic study. This episode required ventricular stimulation for several minutes until 1:1 conduction was reestablished.

Branch blocks or hemiblocks in the ECG in patients with CChC are consistent with diffuse lesions in which neither focal nor complete disruption of the structures is seen.[7] The bundle block in the ECG arises as a result of better conduction through the least affected branch. Nevertheless, evidence of complete disruption of one or more branches can sometimes be obtained, and a real monofascicular system of intraventricular conduction may be discovered. This phenomenon is shown in Figure 11-3, an intracavitary recording in a patient with RBBB and left anterior hemiblock. There is Mobitz I AV block with Wenckebach periodicity during atrial stimulation. Analysis of this tracing confirms that the location of Mobitz I is intraventricular, that is, in the posterior division.

Bradycardia- or tachycardia-dependent intraventricular conduction disturbances are also seen frequently. In Figure 11-4, complete AV block developed in a patient with 2:1 intraventricular block at rest during rapid pacing. AV block may develop in some patients after a long HH interval due to sinus bradycardia following a compensatory pause of either atrial or ventricular premature beats (Fig. 11-5).

Some pharmacologic tests have been useful in unmasking latent conduction disturbances. Chiale et al.[19] induced significant conduction

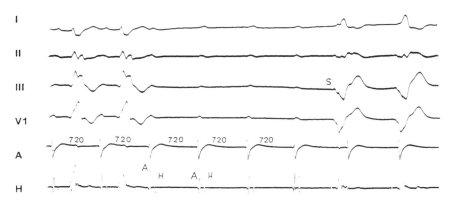

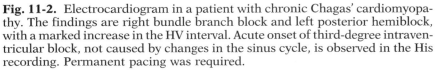

Fig. 11-2. Electrocardiogram in a patient with chronic Chagas' cardiomyopathy. The findings are right bundle branch block and left posterior hemiblock, with a marked increase in the HV interval. Acute onset of third-degree intraventricular block, not caused by changes in the sinus cycle, is observed in the His recording. Permanent pacing was required.

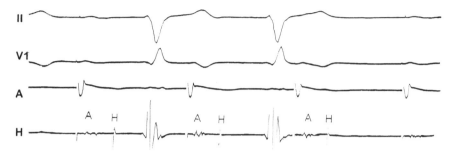

Fig. 11-3. Severe disturbances of intraventricular conduction in a patient with chronic Chagas' cardiomyopathy. In the His recording, intraventricular conduction is considerably lengthened during atrial pacing (S1-S2 = 730 msec), with an intraventricular Wenckebach block (Mobitz I) in the posterior division. This event is caused by a monofascicular conduction system (right bundle branch block and left anterior hemiblock).

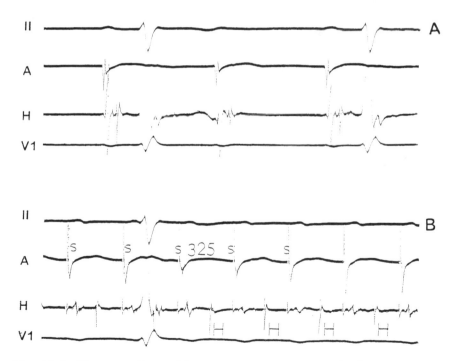

Fig. 11-4. Electrocardiographic tracings in a patient with chronic Chagas' cardiomyopathy. *Upper panel,* Tracing demonstrates right bundle branch block and left anterior hemiblock. The His recording shows a 2:1 infra-His block. *Lower panel,* During rapid atrial pacing, complete infra-His block was induced.

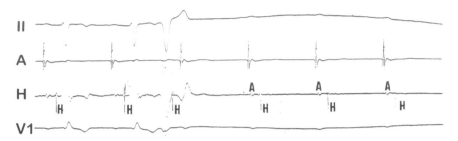

Fig. 11-5. Electrocardiogram in a patient with chronic Chagas' cardiomyopathy, right bundle branch block, and left anterior hemiblock. A ventricular premature beat with retrograde conduction through the His bundle induces a long HH interval (1,400 msec), triggering complete intraventricular block.

disturbances in the right bundle branch and in the anterior division of the left bundle with ajmaline, a depressant of intraventricular conduction in patients with CChC and normal ECG findings. The response to pharmacologic testing is usually more conspicuous in patients with previously noted incomplete RBBB. However, these findings should be considered carefully, because they consist of a nonspecific response that can also be triggered in persons without CChC.

Conclusions

Bradyarrhythmias in Chagas' disease frequently have a different meaning than in other cardiomyopathies, although management is similar. Patients with CChC may harbor conduction disturbances for long periods of time, although these alterations are sometimes independent of the clinical course.

Bundle branch blocks, either isolated or associated with sinus bradycardia, are of early onset and have a slow evolution, during which no other clinical findings, such as cardiac dilatation and hemodynamic failure, may be seen. Whether complete AV block develops is unpredictable, varying greatly from one individual to another. This feature makes it possible for patients to remain asymptomatic for a long time, even several years, until the sudden appearance of ventricular arrhythmias or heart failure, which swiftly changes the course of the disease.

The indication for a pacemaker is related to the severity of arrhythmia whether the patient does or does not have symptoms. Nevertheless, malignant ventricular arrhythmias requiring antiarrhythmic drugs that may depress the conduction system and hemodynamic failure associated with chronotropic incompetence may be clear indications for pacing, even without AV block.

A well-known concept among health care workers who frequently treat patients with Chagas' disease is "Chagasic patients can withstand arrhythmias better than others can." This observation is validated by the fact that in other cardiomyopathies, the arrhythmias are the result of an anatomical and functional injury to the heart, whereas in Chagas' disease, they appear long before anatomical damage to and dilatation of the myocardium and hemodynamic failure.

References

1. Chagas C: Processos patojenicos da tripanosomiase americana. Mem Inst Oswaldo Cruz viii:5-36, 1916
2. Rosenbaum MB: Chagasic cardiomyopathy. Prog Cardiovasc Dis 7:199-225, 1964
3. Rassi A, Carneiro O: Estudio clinico electrocardiografico e radiologico da cardiopatia chagasica cronica. Analise de 106 casos. Rev Goiania Med 2:287-307, 1956
4. Laranja FS, Dias E, Nobrega G, Miranda A: Chagas' disease; a clinical, epidemiologic, and pathologic study. Circulation 14:1035-1060, 1956
5. Andrade ZA, Andrade SG, Oliveira GB, Alonso DR: Histopathology of the conducting tissue of the heart in Chagas' myocarditis. Am Heart J 95:316-324, 1978
6. Storino R, Milci J: Enfermedad de Chagas. Doyma Argentina Ed, 1994, pp 141-183
7. Andrade ZA: Aspectos patológicos da doenca de Chagas. Interciencia 8:367, 1983
8. Hernández-Pieretti O, Lozano-Wilson JR, Urbina-Quintana A, Villoria G, de Hernández MI, Gómez-Amundarain E: Sick sinus syndrome in chronic Chagas' heart disease (abstract). Am J Cardiol 33:144, 1974
9. Andrade ZA, Camara EJ, Sadigursky M, Andrade SG: Sinus node involvement in Chagas' disease [Portuguese]. Arq Bras Cardiol 50:153-158, 1988
10. Thery C, Gosselin B, Lekieffre J, Warembourg H: Pathology of sinoatrial node. Correlations with electrocardiographic findings in 111 patients. Am Heart J 93:735-740, 1977
11. Mott KE, Hagstrom JWC: The pathologic lesions of the cardiac autonomic nervous system in chronic Chagas' myocarditis. Circulation 31:273-286, 1965
12. Köberle F: Über das neurotoxin des *Trypanosoma cruzi*. Zentralbl Allg Path 95:486, 1956
13. Caeiro T, Iosa D: Chronic Chagas' disease: possible mechanism of sinus bradycardia. Can J Cardiol 10:765-768, 1994
14. Junqueira Junior LF, Beraldo PS, Chapadeiro E, Jesus PC: Cardiac autonomic dysfunction and neuroganglionitis in a rat model of chronic Chagas' disease. Cardiovasc Res 26:324-329, 1992
15. Elizari MV, Chiale PA, Del Negro B: Arritmias en la enfermedad de Chagas. *In* Actualizaciones en la Enfermedad de Chagas. Edited by RJ Madoery, C Madoery, MI Cámara. Buenos Aires, Organismo Oficial del Congreso Nacional Medicina, 1993, pp 215-227
16. Anselmi A, Gurdiel O, Suarez JA, Anselmi G: Disturbances in the A-V conduction system in Chagas' myocarditis in the dog. Circ Res 20:56-64, 1967
17. Rosenbaum MB, Alvarez AJ: Electrocardiogram in chronic chagasic myocarditis. Am Heart J 50:492-527, 1955

18. Rosenbaum MB, Elizari MV, Lázzari JO, Kretz A, da Ruos HO: The clinical causes and mechanisms of intraventricular conduction disturbances. *In* Advances in Electrocardiography. Edited by RC Schlant, JW Hurst. New York, Grune & Stratton, 1972, pp 183-220

19. Chiale PA, Przybylski J, Laino RA, Halpern MS, Sanchez RA, Gabrieli A, Elizari MV, Rosenbaum MB: Electrocardiographic changes evoked by ajmaline in chronic Chagas' disease with manifest myocarditis. Am J Cardiol 49:14-20, 1982

Index

AAALDK (myosin-specific epitope), 21
Acute Chagas' disease, 28-32
AIDS (acquired immunodeficiency syndrome), 45
Amiodarone, 102, 104-109
Angiography, 42
Antiarrhythmic drugs, 101-109
Antiparasite response, 21-22
Arrhythmias
    atrial, 110-111
    pharmacologic treatment, 95-112
    signal-averaged electrocardiography predictors, 77-79
    ventricular, 97-110
Arrhythmogenic substrate, 79-80
Arterial baroreceptor sensitivity, 57-58
Atrial arrhythmias, 110-111
Atrioventricular block, 84-88
Atrioventricular node, 146
Autoimmunity, 21-22
Autonomic nervous system, 98-99

Blood tests, 36
Bradyarrhythmias, 84-88, 143-151
    atrioventricular node, 146
    bundle of His, 146-147

left and right bundle branches, 143, 147-150
    myocarditis, 144-145
    sinoatrial node, 145-146
Bradycardia-tachycardia syndrome, 84
Bundle of His, 146-147

Cardiac autonomic reflex function, 51-64
    anatomical alterations, 52-53
    in Chagas' cardiomyopathy, 54-59
    pathophysiology, 53-54
    and treatment of Chagas' cardioneuropathy, 59, 62
Cardiac catheterization. See Catheterization
Cardiac rate. See Heart rate
Cardiomyopathy, 34-36
    bradyarrhythmias in, 143-151
    cardiac reflex function in, 54-59
    clinical characteristics of patients with, 131-133
    and signal-averaged electrocardiography, 71
Cardioneuropathy, 59, 62
Catheter ablation, 123-125
    with alcohol, 123
    radiofrequency, 89, 123-124

153

transthoracic epicardial, 124-125

Catheterization, cardiac, 42

Chagas' disease
acute, 28-32
chronic, 11-12, 34-36, 95-112
classification of, 37-41
clinical aspects of, 27-47
clinical relevance of invasive
electrophysiologic studies,
83-91
effects on cardiac autonomic
reflex function, 51-64
etiology of, 5-6
final stage, 44-45
implantable cardioverter-defibrillator use in, 129-140
indeterminate phase, 32-33
molecular pathology of, 19-23
pathophysiology of, 6-7
signal-averaged electrocardiography in, 71-79
in U.S., 1-2
ventricular tachycardia in,
117-126
See also Heart disease, Chagas'; Trypanosoma cruzi

Chemotherapy, 12-13

Chronic Chagas' disease, 11-12,
34-36, 95-112

Circadian rhythm, of sustained
ventricular tachyarrhythmias,
137,
139-140

Class I antiarrhythmic drugs,
101, 102-109

Class II antiarrhythmic drugs,
102

Class III antiarrhythmic drugs,
102-109

Class IV antiarrhythmic drugs,
102-109

Cloned parasite antigens, 19-20

Cold pressor test, 56-57

Coronary artery disease, 135,
137

Differential diagnosis, 45, 46

Drugs. See Pharmacologic treatment; specific drugs

ECG. See Electrocardiography

Echocardiography, 30-31, 40-41

Electrocardiography (ECG), 29-30, 33, 37, 39
See also Signal-averaged electrocardiography

Electrophysiologically guided resection, 119-120

Electrophysiologic studies, 83-91
in bradyarrhythmias, 84-88
in tachyarrhythmias, 88-90

ELISA (enzyme-linked immunosorbent assay), 8-19

Endomyocardial biopsy, 43

Epidemiology, 28

Fast Fourier transform, 68, 74

Frequency domain technique,
68, 70, 74, 77-78, 79

Heart disease, Chagas'
acute, 29-31
control and treatment, 47
pharmacologic treatment of arrhythmias in chronic, 95-112
severe, 20-21
in U.S., 1-3
See also Cardiomyopathy

Heart rate
response, 54-55
variability, 59
and ventricular arrhythmias,
98-99

Implantable cardioverter-defibrillator, 111-112, 129-140

in Chagas' disease and coronary artery disease, 135, 137
in chagasic cardiomyopathy patients, 131-133
clinical outcome, 133-134
complications, 134
evaluation before implantation, 130-131
mortality with, 134
time of first shock, 135, 137
Invasive electrophysiologic studies, 83-91

Late potentials, 68
Left bundle branch block, 143, 147-150
Low frequency to high frequency index, 59, 61

Metoprolol, 62, 63
Mexiletine, 102, 104, 109
Molecular diagnostic methods, 10-11
Molecular pathology, 19-23
17-Monochloroacetylajmaline, 102, 104
Myocardial infarction, 70-71
Myocarditis, 20-21, 144-145

Natural history, 27, 34-35
Neurologic disease, 32

Ophthalmolymphangitis complex, 29
Orthostatic stress, 55-56

Pacing, 134, 135, 136
Parasite intracellular proteins, 20-21
Paroxysmal sustained ventricular tachyarrhythmia, 88
Pathogenesis, 28

Pharmacologic treatment
of ventricular arrhythmias, 101-109
See also specific drugs

Radiofrequency catheter ablation, 89, 123-124
Radionuclide angiography, 42
Right bundle branch block, 143, 147-150
Risk factors, 45, 47
Romaña's eye sign, 29

Scintigraphy, 42
Signal-averaged electrocardiography, 67-80
in Chagas' disease, 71-79
methods, 72-74
after myocardial infarction, 70-71
in patients with cardiomyopathies, 71
as predictor of arrhythmic events, 77-79
prevalence of abnormalities on, 74-77
recording techniques, 68-70
Sinoatrial node, 145-146
Sinus bradycardia, 54
Sinus node, 110-111
Sodium channel blocking agents, 104
d,l-Sotalol, 109
Spectral turbulence analysis technique, 74
Sudden death, 45, 108
Surgery
anatomically guided, 120, 122-123
electrophysiologically guided resection, 119-120
Sustained ventricular tachyarrhythmias, 137, 139-140

Tachyarrhythmias, 88-90, 137, 139-140

Time domain technique, 68, 69, 78

Total power spectra, 59, 60

Transthoracic epicardial ablation, 124-125

Trypanosoma cruzi
blood tests for, 36
cloned antigens, 19
diagnosis of, 7-11
epidemiology, 28
genome project, 22-23
markers for follow-up of chemotherapy, 12-13
pathogenesis, 28
transmission of, 5-6
in U.S., 1-2

Trypanosoma rangeli, 11

Valsalva maneuver, 56

Ventricular arrhythmias, 97-110
autonomic nervous system and cardiac rate, 98-99
electrophysiologic mechanisms, 100-101
nonconventional medical treatment, 109-110
pharmacologic treatment, 101-109
potentially malignant, 97-98, 100, 108

Ventricular tachyarrhythmias, 137, 139-140

Ventricular tachycardia, 117-126

Verapamil, 102-104